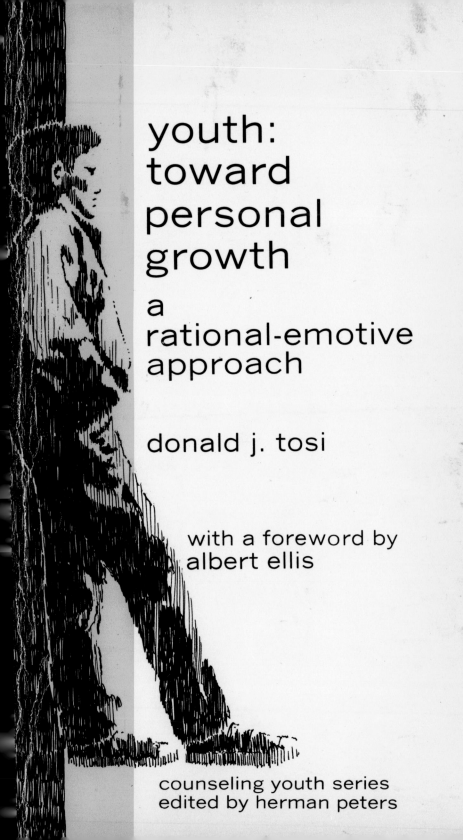

youth:
toward
personal
growth

a
rational-emotive
approach

donald j. tosi

with a foreword by
albert ellis

counseling youth series
edited by herman peters

* youth: toward personal growth

a rational-emotive approach

donald j. tosi

the ohio state university

charles e. merrill publishing company
a bell & howell company
columbus, ohio 43216

✳ counseling youth series

under the editorship of

herman peters
the ohio state university

published by
charles e. merrill publishing company
a bell & howell company
columbus, ohio 43216

*International Standard Book
Number*:   0-675-08877-1

*Library of Congress Catalog
Card Number*:   73-86023

Printed in the United
States of America

foreword

Although many articles and books have been written about rational-emotive therapy (RET), this is the first full presentation that is specifically directed to young peope, and I think that it is a notable addition to the therapeutic literature.

As is the case with various other kinds of counseling and psychotherapy, there are several sources of widespread confusion about RET. This is perhaps because it is a comprehensive, cognitive-emotive-behavioral system, and some presenters and interpreters emphasize one of its major aspects to the neglect of one or more of its other major components. I myself have sometimes overstressed its rational-persuasive side, partly because it is one of the few therapeutic schools that concretly points out what individuals say to themselves to make themselves upset or disturbed and how their internalized cognitions can be quickly seen, logically analyzed, and empirically disconfirmed when they are self-defeating. I consequently first called RET *rational psychotherapy*, to distinguish it from other methodologies.

That title led to some serious misunderstandings, since RET is also highly emotive-evocative and behavioral. On the emotive side, rational-emotive therapists forcefully confront clients, use down-to-earth language, give full nonblaming acceptance (or what Carl Rogers calls "unconditional positive regard"), use many encounter exercises, evoke suppressed feelings, employ rational-emotive imagery (REI), and utilize various other dramatic techniques. On the behavioral side, they almost always give activity homework assignments (akin to *in vivo* desensitization), teach assertive training, do modeling and behavioral rehearsal, employ operant conditioning, and use a variety of other methods. RET, therefore, could easily be called something like rational-emotive-behavior therapy (REBT) or rational behavior therapy (RBT), and some of its adherents, particularly Dr. Maxie C. Maultsby, Jr., frequently use the latter term.

Fortunately, Professor Tosi exposits, in this book, a wide range of rational-emotive procedures, and he shows young people how they can be specifically applied to their own emotional problems. He also, much to my own satisfaction, points out some of the most humanistic bases and procedures of RET. As I have tried to show in my book, *Humanistic Psychotherapy: The Rational-Emotive Approach* (New York: Julian Press, 1973), RET is one of the most humanistically oriented systems of understanding and changing personality. For it solidly begins with values and assumes that practically all men and women *value* (or give importance to) surviving, being relatively happy, living successfully in a social community, and relating intimately to a few selected others. They *choose* these goals, and when they are rational or sane, they choose to abet them; when they are irrational or disturbed, they choose to sabotage them. RET teaches them how to be more happily human by giving up their unrealistic demands to be superhuman and their almost inevitable concomitant conclusions that they are subhuman.

Professor Tosi shows his readers how they can use RET to stop deceiving themselves, to fully accept their humanity, to actualize their potentials for happy living, and to act more authentically to achieve the goals that they can choose and achieve.

Albert Ellis, Ph.D.

*institute for advanced study in
rational psychotherapy
new york, new york*

consulting editor's foreword

Since the early 1900s, when G. Stanley Hall acknowledged the developmental stage of "adolescence"—the teens—the sequence of development has been from adolescence to adulthood. However with the many cultural changes in recent years, there has emerged a new stage—youth. Certainly the persons in the range of eighteen to thirty years are far beyond the characteristic immaturity associated with adolescence. On the other hand, these youth are not ready for many of the commitments associated with adulthood.

In a very real way, youth is the period of pristine freedom, and legal, ethical, cultural, technological, and work exploration is being done during this period. The options are there. Thus, if there were ever a developmental stage in need of counseling and guidance services, it is the period of youth. Because of the residue of adolescence, the new freedoms, the demands for gaining maturity, and the conflicts of "first" freedoms, many youth can and do profit from counseling.

The confusion and irrationality of this transitional period lends itself to the bent of rational-emotive counseling. My colleague, Donald J. Tosi, presents in this book an excellent introduction for counselors using a rational-emotive approach with youth.

Rational-emotive counseling has gained considerable merit as a way of counseling youth. Its rational development, affective options, and "homework" possibilities offer youth a wide range of activities for enhancing behaviors and eliminating self-defeating behaviors. The confrontation, and "down-to-earth-to-man" relationships of the developmental stage of youth gives a foundation for effective counseling. The wide range of rational-emotive procedures is another "plus" in counseling youth. It is especially appropriate for many of today's alienated youth because RET implies that the young person is "valued" and can search for better ways to improve.

The examples contained in this text are reality based. Too many counseling protocols seem like anemic conversations with "niceness" the undergirding technique, although the real world rarely operates this way—despite hundreds of years of effort to make it truly human.

This book will be of use to counselors, but not to be overlooked is its usefulness for many guidance-oriented teachers who work with students. In addition, as Dr. Ellis notes in his foreword, it is a "first" in its field. The author is authentic. The counseling procedures are "for real" structures in the mid and late 1970s. For many readers, the content of this book will be a "good fit" in helping their counseling of youth to become authentic.

Herman J. Peters

preface

Rational-emotive counseling is a humanistic approach to the many problems and dilemmas of man's existence. Unlike other systems of counseling
that have been preoccupied with a strict, biological, or environmental
interpretation and explanation of the human phenomenon, rational-
emotive theory (Ellis, 1970) places man in the center of the universe
and of his own fate. Moreover, man is seen as having almost full responsibility for choosing and creating his own existence. In spite of the many
biological and early environmental influences that limit him and which
are obviously operative in his present behavior, man has the ability to
intervene significantly between environmental inputs and his emotional-
behavioral outputs. Rational-emotive theory brings into focus the importance of man's remarkable ability to engage in high-level cognitive
or thought processes. The theory also emphasizes that it is precisely man's
capability to think rationally and/or creatively that separates him from
other animals and allows him to do something about the numerous biological, environmental, and social forces that tend to dehumanize him.
    The system could be labeled easily as a solely cognitive therapy,
but this would be unfair. As we shall see later, rational-emotive theory
and technique consider the whole person. As a system, rational-emotive
theory attends to the cognitive, the affective, and the behavioral-motoric
growth of the person. Concommitantly, RE theory emphasizes the importance of the person's environment and his interaction with that
environment.
    A variety of intervention strategies are employed by practicing
rational-emotive counselors. Some of these strategies have derived from

behavioristic methods which emphasize operant conditioning, classical conditioning, and social modeling. Others, which attend to affective processes, have been derived from Freudian psychoanalysis and the so-called nondirective or relationship-oriented therapies. But the set of techniques and methods which stresses cognition and is unique to rational-emotive theory will be described later in this book.

In this text, rational-emotive counseling will be explored as it applies to a number of the concerns expressed by today's youth culture. Youth, defined as persons between the ages of sixteen and thirty, will not be depicted as a psychologically superior group who are more "together," more "human," more "feeling," or more "with it" than are other age groups. They will be treated as persons who face many of the same human dilemmas that persons in other age groups face. Whenever possible, I have tried to ignore the usual symbols that prevent persons from knowing, accepting, and acting towards others in reasonable ways. By attending to the personal meanings ascribed to symbols, I have found that persons have much in common, especially in the way in which they go about defeating their own existence and disturbing themselves needlessly.

A counselor can encounter his client effectively only when he recognizes and fully understands the client's personal definition of himself and the world in which he interacts. That is, to a significant extent, the counselor needs to be attuned to the client's internalized meanings, values, and beliefs. In a counseling relationship, constructive changes in clients are more likely to occur if the counselor confronts his clients actively, directly, openly, and honestly with their self-defeating ways of thinking, believing, and behaving and then proceeds to teach them the ways and means of acquiring a more self-enhancing set of meanings, beliefs, values, and behaviors—or, more specifically, a self-enhancing personal philosophy.

The specific concepts and techniques of RE counseling with youth will be presented in the forthcoming chapters. The first chapter includes a descriptive model for human growth, developmental factors, parameters of the counseling process, and aims or goals of counseling. The second chapter presents rational-emotive philosophy and concepts. The third chapter describes Ellis's ten irrational ideas and their rational alternatives. Chapter four deals with the use of specific techniques in rational-emotive counseling, singly and in combination with techniques derived from other schools of thoughts. The fifth chapter consists of transcripts of rational-emotive encounters which depict the struggles of youth. The last chapter, although brief, focuses upon rational-emotive group counseling and guidance.

Donald J. Tosi

author's note

To be able to think about oneself or to be conscious of one's consciousness may be man's most prized human possession. For its is this facility that separates man from other animals. It is precisely this unique activity which allows one to transcend the biological and sociological influences that too often encapsulate him. Rational-emotive counseling and psychotherapy, though directive, authoritative and even sometimes bold, aim at developing in man the capacity he has to grow in thought, feeling, and action. In other words, it aims to free man to think and act for himself in the world in which he lives. Rational-emotive theory assumes that until man is free to know, to accept, and to affirm himself, he cannot fully know, accept, or affirm others.

It should be clear at the outset that rational-emotive theory and practice do not determine how one will create himself or what he ultimately becomes. That rational-emotive counseling is largely devoid of mysticism, metaphor, and poetry is humanly realistic. Perhaps the major goal of rational-emotive counseling is to minimize the person's self-distorting and self-deceiving tendencies so that he may ultimately live more authentically. To achieve such an end, the counselor himself must freely enter into a working alliance with his client in which a "cognitive reconstruction or reorganization of the self" becomes a distinct possibility for the client.

Donald J. Tosi

acknowledgements

I must extend great appreciation to many colleagues, graduate students, and professional clients for their assistance in developing this manuscript. My close friend, colleague, and mentor Dr. Joseph Quaranta has helped me conceptualize the essential parameters of personal growth, and I have found the ideas of Dr. Ross Mooney and Dr. Quaranta extremely useful in looking at rational-emotive theory and counseling from a slightly different perspective.

I am also indebted to Dr. Albert Ellis for taking time to write the foreword to this book. His writings have pervaded my own teaching, writing, and practice of counseling and psychotherapy, not to mention my personal life.

To Dr. William A. Carlson, I am grateful, for Dr. Carlson, a former colleague of mine at Western Michigan University, encouraged me as a counseor and therapist. More than my colleague, Bill also was my teacher and is still a close friend.

I also appreciate the assistance given me by several of my students. Dr. Richard Moleski and Sharon Seggerson provided some of the case material in chapter four. Their assistance in preparing this chapter was invaluable.

Herman J. Peters, a friend and colleague at the Ohio State University, made the publication of this manuscript a very rewarding experience for me. Dr. Peters' comments and ideas are appreciated.

Karen Storts typed the drafts of this manuscript. To her, I am also indebted. Others who have directly or indirectly assisted me are too numerous to mention, but Dr. Gilbert Mazer, Dr. M.E. Wilson, Dr. Edna Menke, Dr. R.F. Frumkin, and Dr. Larry Litwack are some who cannot go unmentioned.

I am grateful to my wife, Josie, and my two daughters, Francesca and Nicole. Their patience, love, and understanding made the writing of this book possible. I hope the contents of this manuscript will have strong implications for the personal growth of my two daughters and, certainly, for our family.

Finally, my deepest appreciation goes to my parents, Henry and Rose Tosi. My father passed away during the final phase of production of this manuscript. To him, I am deeply indepted. From both of my parents I have derived some of my deepest understandings of myself and others. In fact, I may have learned one of the most basic tenets of REC from them—self-acceptance for I have learned that in spite of what a person does, he is always of value—at least to himself.

———

contents

one ✳ human development and counseling: parameters

a model for personal growth

In our attempt to understand people, it is very useful to have some model or framework that allows us to attend to the relevant personal and environmental factors associated with man's growth and development. The model should specify parameters and while it should not limit our description of the human organism or create any bias, it should, at the same time, guide our efforts. Mooney (1963) has provided such a model which he terms "self in situation" or "person in environment" (Quaranta, 1971; Tosi, 1971).

Mooney's model (see Figure 1) depicts a person as having three essential, but interrelated components or processes which are cognitive, affective, and behavioral in nature. Developmentally, they center around the knowledge, acceptance, and affirmation of the self within the world in which the individual lives. Specifically, the model portrays a person who thinks, feels, and acts within a socio-cultural system. This person does not grow or develop cognitively, affectively, or behaviorally in isolation from other persons or things. His growth and development depend upon the manner in which he interacts with his environment and upon the way his environment interacts with him. The infinity sign in Figure 1 designates the reciprocal relationship between man and his environment. The person's environment is viewed as being the number

1

of possible situations the person encounters. For instance, an environment would consist of persons, institutions, physical and material things, or any combination of these items. The family, the school, the peer group, the job, and their respective facets and ramifications are some of the significant environments in which the person operates.

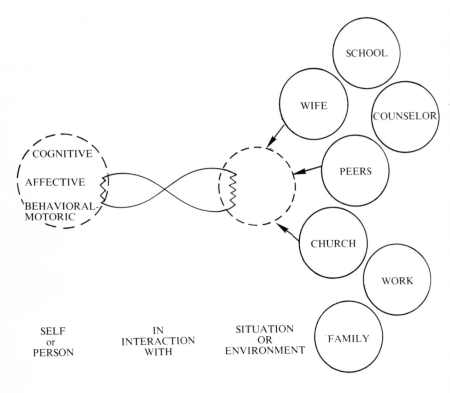

SELF or PERSON   IN INTERACTION WITH   SITUATION OR ENVIRONMENT

figure one

the model

In the first phase of human development, the infant's behavior is dominated primarily by emotional or affective processes, for his cognitive functions are only in the incipient stage. His crying, for instance, is the result of tension caused by hunger, thirst, or other physical irritation. On the other hand, the infant becomes quiescent when his physical needs have been satisfied. As man interacts further with his environment, an elaborate set of cognitive functions emerge which enable him to achieve greater control and mastery over his feelings, actions, and environments. These cognitive processes encompass his ability to think or reflect upon himself and his environment, to solve problems, to think creatively, to abstract, and to evaluate himself and his environment. Man's facility to appraise, to interpret, and to ascribe evaluative labels to his behavior and/or his feelings gives, in large measure, meaning to his affective-behavioral states. In addition, evaluative thinking is fundamental to man's system of valuing and believing.

Man's actions in relation to his environment are often met with consequences from that environment. Sometimes, these consequences may be of such a nature that they do not permit man to develop himself most effectively. In other words, while a person may be capable of assessing accurately his feelings about his environment, he may lack many of the specific behavioral-motoric skills which would enable him to act more efficiently upon that environment.

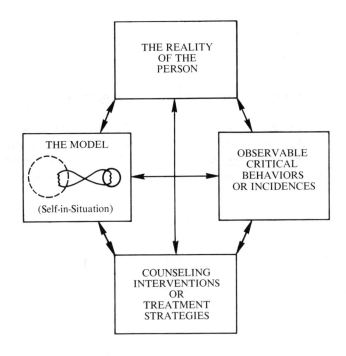

figure two

a conceptual framework*

*J. Quaranta, "Conceptual Framework for Career Development Programming," in *Guidance and Evaluative Career Development*, ed. R. McCormick and J. Wigtil. Project sponsored by Division of Guidance and Testing. (Columbus: Ohio Department of Education, 1971).

Cognitive, affective, and behavioral processes all operate in a unitary fashion as man interacts with his environment. These functions are considered temporarily apart from each other as discrete functions only to facilitate an understanding of the whole person. The "person-in-environment" model tells us what to look for in persons as they grow and develop in environments. The model provides parameters of growth and attends to cognitive, affective, behavioral, and social areas. In a sense, as do most models, it attends to "what should be."

As counselors, we need to have an accurate way of describing and understanding our client's world. We must be certain that our intervention strategies are appropriate to that world. Furthermore, it is necessary to be able to observe that critical experiences and behaviors have occurred in the client's life following our specific interventions. A conceptual framework which depicts the relationship between the client's real world, the model, the intervention strategies, and critical experiences or behaviors is provided in Figure 2. Ideally, there is a convergence of these factors in counseling.

developmental processes

Youth often express feelings of alienation, despair, hopelessness, and misunderstanding. Moreover, they often complain of a lack of meaning in their lives and of feeling little relevance in the present-day society. In short, youth often feel alone in their struggle for meaning and relevancy and, concomitantly, often lack trust in adults.

While it is normal and, perhaps, even natural for most persons to experience these conditions, many persons fail to grow beyond such attitudes by perpetuating them in thought and action. For many of our youth, the striving for meaning and relevance is often an inauthentic, neurotic, self-defeating process which is masked by contemporary symbols such as the drug culture, the Jesus movement, women's lib, or gay lib—to mention only a few. In this section, consideration will be given to the developmental stages that precede and include the period defined as youth (sixteen to thirty years of age). The intent of depicting the individual's development from early childhood to adulthood is to highlight those human processes that are growth enhancing and those that are growth inhibiting Lidy (1968).

infancy (birth to eighteen months)

The period of infancy is usually defined somewhat arbitrarily as the first eighteen months of the child's life. During this period, the infant is almost totally helpless and dependent upon his parents, especially his mother, for gratification of his needs. The infant spends the greater part of his time sleeping. His innate response to frustration is one of the most basic mechanisms of survival, crying. When he is hungry, the child usually signals his mother by crying seemingly incessantly until she responds by placing the nipple of her breast or the bottle into his mouth and his excitement subsides.

The infancy period is characterized by profound growth—physical-motoric, affective, and cognitive. Piaget (1953) labels this stage of cognitive growth the "sensorimotor period." While cognitive development originates in simple reflexive behavior and is initially dependent upon experience and maturation, the child progressively achieves more control over his movements which enables him to interact with, assimilate, and accommodate more features of his environment to himself. Through trial-and-error processes or random exploration, the child gradually learns about his environment and shows some incipient signs of mastering certain aspects of it. The child gradually develops an internal, primitive, mental imagery which he uses in problem-solving. During this period, the child perceives himself as an object of actions, while, at the same time, showing signs of differentiating himself from the environment.

Cognitive and emotional growth occur simultaneously within specific environmental situations. If the environments which nurture human growth are self-inhibiting (in the sense that they deny the infant his natural tendencies toward growth in all three areas of self), the infant will experience states of excessive frustration and tension which will impede or obstruct this movement through later developmental stages.

Erikson (1968) has postulated that the most critical task of infancy involves the child's development of the rudiments of basic trust or confidence in himself and others. If the mother is reasonably dependable in her care of the child and exudes confidence and security in herself, the child is likely to assume some of these basic traits. If, on the other hand, the mother is highly anxious, pays too little or too much attention to the child, and is generally inconsistent in her behavior, the child is likely to develop a sense of insecurity or mistrust. Unusual deprivation of the child's physiological and safety needs during the infancy period arouses frustration and anxiety which can lead to the later development of fears and suspicions about the world and, more specifically, other people.

infancy (eighteen months to three years)

When the child emerges from the stages of early infancy and begins to walk and talk, he enters another crucial period of development. It is during the second and third years of his development that he is exposed more often to the realities of socialization. The child must learn to delay the immediate gratification of some of his most basic needs, such as elimination and hunger. In other words, he is taught by his parents and others the value of becoming a long-term "hedonist" as opposed to a short-term "hedonist." Essentially, the young child must develop a healthy ego which will keep some of his normal biological tendencies in balance.

The child is expected to become less dependent upon his mother and more dependent upon himself during this period. Erickson (1968) identifies this period as one in which the child develops greater mastery over his environment and establishes autonomy as opposed to shame and doubt. In addition, there is rapid language and conceptual development as the child develops simple systems of ascribing meanings to his cultural environment.

Many conflicts between the child and his parents are in evidence during this period. The attitudes and values of the mother and father are communicated in a variety of social exchanges. For instance, if the parents are excessively anxious about sexual activities, this anxiety may be transmitted to the child through verbal or physical punishment for the child's natural sexual tendencies, such as in the normal pleasure he derives from manipulating his genitals or his bowel and urinary movements. In response to the frustrations he experiences, the child may counteract by withholding his feces or simply rejecting many of his parent's demands. He also may acquire a foundation of such self-defeating emotions as shame and self-doubt. His experience of these self-defeating emotions may be perpetuated throughout his life unless he is exposed to other situations that pose alternative conditions of a more positive nature.

Assuming he has been exposed to reasonable parental child-rearing practices, the child will manifest a sense of accomplishment and self-assurance in his behavior when he emerges from this second stage. Moreover, he will begin to demonstrate an ability to delay the immediate gratification of some of his basic needs in favor of a time that is more appropriate for their expression. The child at this age shows remarkable control over his motor behavior. He initiates many of his own activities, imitates the behavior of others, and shows much progress in language development and use of his imagination.

In his cognitive growth, the child reaches a level during this period in which he begins to systematize his knowledge about physical and social events, to construct logical structures, and to reconstruct the practical knowledge he has gained during the sensorimotor period. The child, egocentrically, believes everyone thinks the same things he does;

he never questions his cognitions as he thinks these are the only possible ones and he therefore must be correct. Piaget refers to this cognitive stage as the "preoperational period" of intelligence. The preoperational period also pervades the third stage of development which, for our purposes, we will call early childhood.

early childhood (three-and-a-half to five years)

The period of early childhood is characterized by the child's mastery over his body. He begins to initiate many of his own activities and shows much progress in language development and the use of imagery. Erickson (1968) suggests that the child must learn to maintain a balance between initiative and guilt during this time. Initiative involves the identification of the child with the parents in his attempt to acquire their love and approval. If parents discriminately reward the child for his self-initiated activities or appropriate sex-role behaviors, the child is likely to increase the probability of making initiating responses. Parents reinforce initiative in their children when they attend to the child's questions or inquiries; conversely, if the child is indiscriminantly rewarded or punished for appropriate sex-role initiative responses, he is likely to develop a sense of guilt or self-depreciation over his initiative behavior. If no change occurs in the negative responses of the parents, the child will have a greater tendency to maintain these self-defeating tendencies in later developmental stages. The degree to which the child learns guilt and self-depreciation behaviors during this period serves as the basis for deep-seated feelings of inferiority that may emerge during the stage of middle childhood.

middle childhood (six to eleven years)

The period of middle childhood is often characterized as the latency sexual period. Erickson (1968) believes that the psycho-social bipolarity which emerges during this time is industry vs. inferiority. Early in the period, the child enters a new and significant social situation—the school—where his environment is expanded and new interpersonal relationships with peers and teachers develop. Especially apparent is the tendency of boys and girls to identify with peers and significant adults of the same sex. Many essential social traits develop out of the child's interactions with his peers, and the child's peer group becomes of the utmost importance to him.

In terms of cognitive development, the child makes the transition from the period of preoperational thought to the period of concrete operations during which logical thought patterns begin to emerge slowly. Essentially, the period of concrete operations involves the child's use of systematic reasoning about various situational events—real and imagined. The child realizes that other individuals can have beliefs and ideas which are different from his, thus making it necessary for him to validate his own thoughts. At this juncture, however, according to Inhelder and Piaget, the child does not carry out formal operations which involve thinking in propositions, hypotheses, and abstract reasoning (1958).

During these elementary-school years, or period of middle childhood, the child makes an effort to participate in many industrious activities, which might include sewing, fishing, cooking, drawing, and painting. Again, if parents, teachers, and other significant individuals encourage the child in these new behaviors through positive reinforcement, he is likely to perpetuate industrious behavior in later years. When the child is physically punished or ignored for performing industrious activities, he will probably develop rather intense feelings of inferiority.

As the child develops cognitively, he makes increasing use of verbal symbols to label internal and external events. He develops an awareness and a concept of self. More than ever before, he attaches verbal symbols to those negative emotional conditions which we have been calling guilt, doubt, and inferiority. It is as though the child now says to himself, when his parent beats or rejects him for initiating some activity, "I am bad. I am not good like my brother or big sister." Such sentences or verbal cues become attached to those negative emotional states and then serve to mediate cognitively events occurring outside the child and his internal affective or emotional responses. During this period of development, the child learns to think in terms of causality, but it is difficult for him to reflect upon his own appraisal of events. Thus, when a parent is angry at him (an external event), the child's cognitive or evaluative responses may be that "I am bad" or "I am no good," and the resultant emotional response (an internal event) may be a feeling of dejection. Consequently, the child comes to see the external event as the cause of his emotional response, and this type of thinking is generally reinforced by parents, peers, and other adult models.

The verbal symbols attached to both incipient negative or self-defeating and pleasant or self-enhancing emotional states serve as the foundation for the child's personal belief system and value orientation which emerge as screens or filters through which external phenomena are passed, processed, and evaluated. The verbal symbols, usually in the form of internalized sentences, are used by the child to label all sorts of external events and their relationships to internal events (feelings and emotions).

The development of the person in terms of cognitive, affective, and behavioral processes occurs within a socio-cultural system. The child's first social encounters are usually with his mother, father, and family. A second major encounter is with the school. As the child interacts with them, these social situations influence significantly his beliefs about himself and the world.

The school, for instance, is a major socializing agency. Teachers and classmates, while in many instances supporting the child's already existing beliefs and value systems, often create conditions which contradict them. For example, a child may be accepted completely by his parents when he fails at some task at home. But when he fails at some academic task in the classroom, the teacher may punish him and convey the message that "if he is to be a good student, he can, under no circumstances, fail." Thus, the child may say to himself, "Well, when I fail at home, I am good, but when I fail at school, I am bad. It's terrible to fail at school. Only bad kids or dumb kids fail, because that's what the other kids say, and they know a lot. Maybe the other kids are right; I am dumb."

Thus, the school is another major social system within which the child must learn to understand and function rationally. If his experiences in the home have been such that basic trust, initiative, and industry have been fostered, he at least has a foundation upon which he can build to succeed in school. If the child lacks this foundation, it is to be hoped that the school will provide it; however, the typical school curriculum is not always effective in responding to a child's personal-social development.

adolescence (twelve to eighteen years)

The period of adolescence — the years from age twelve to age eighteen — is characterized by the adolescent's undergoing many physiological and psychological changes which are relative to his social environment. Physiologically, the child enters the period of pubescence during which his sexual capabilities and capacity for procreation come into fruition. Psychologically, through his imagination, fantasies, and overt behavior, the adolescent explores new and different kinds of relationships with the opposite sex. The adolescent's newly developed sexual impulses and emerging sexual attitudes become associated with the opposite sex and take the form of love relationships or deep interpersonal attractions. For the first time, the adolescent may experience the pleasure of autoerotic activities as well as erotic activities with members of the opposite sex. Such activities may involve masturbation, kissing, petting, and premarital sex. In many instances, the pleasure of sexual activities has as its consequence in feelings of guilt and shame which have their origins in events which occurred early in the child's development. Some of these feelings of guilt and shame are expected and occur normally, but, in many instances, these feelings or negative affective states may lead to greater self-defeating behavior.

The cognitive transition from concrete operations to formal operations, which involves abstract and rational thinking, occurs during adolescence. The adolescent is able to perform a variety of mental operations on hypothetical propositions; he is able to entertain alternative courses of action, and he has the ability to think in terms of the consequences of his actions. He shows signs of developing a personal philosophy of life as he now thinks about the nature of man and society, the nature of good and evil, and reflects upon himself in relation to these phenomena. Essentially, the adolescent learns to think rationally and scientifically and develops the capacity to apply this type of thinking to his own sense of self.

Erikson (1968) suggests that when the child enters the adolescent period, he confronts the task of developing a clear sense of identity. The Eriksonian bipolarity at this stage is one of identity vs. role confusion. Assuming that the child enters this period with a strong personal base consisting of trust, autonomy, and initiative, the probability of his developing a healthy sense of ego identity is enhanced. If, however, the child lacks this foundation, his chances for acquiring a reasonable psychosocial identity are minimized. In this case, he is likely to develop a sense of role confusion or experience a crisis in his identity.

young adulthood (eighteen to thirty years)

Young adulthood is the stage of development which is by far the most difficult psychologically and sociologically for youth in Western society, as the young adult is expected to make a myriad of significant life decisions and choices. The most important decisions revolve around his education and career and the selection of a marriage partner. The process of selecting one's productive work and the development of close interpersonal relationships with others are often troubled by difficulty.

One of the most important psycho-social tasks of this period is the development of a sense of interpersonal intimacy as opposed to a sense of interpersonal isolation (Erikson, 1968). Intimacy is a feeling and an experience in which one is able to care for another person. The caring is genuine because it is devoid of the neurotic or self-defeating fears and anxieties associated with losing one's own sense of identity. Intimacy involves mutuality, responsibility, closeness, and commitment (Dreyfus, 1972). It should not be construed as being primarily sexual in nature, nor is it always affirmed by one's sexuality. Often, youth believe that intimacy will occur through sexual activities; however, this usually does not happen. An urgency for intimacy can lead to premature and superficial familiarity and can result in a pseudo-intimacy which is deceptive to one or both individuals (Dreyfus, 1972). In its broadest sense, intimacy means a concern for the other person's growth and development as a human being in his own right, and, most of all, a capacity to express this concern or attitude.

If one's value and belief orientation, as it is expressed in his action, has been based firmly in self-trust, industry, and self-identity, the individual will have a greater capacity for intimacy with others. If not, he will experience a sense of neurotic isolation, of being alone — that is, he will feel incapable of being empathetic and personally involved with others.

The capacity for interpersonal intimacy is essential for individual human growth and development, for one's psychological growth evolves out of interpersonal relationships. However, the person who has a great capacity for interpersonal intimacy also may experience a sense of personal isolation or loneliness. This personal isolation or loneliness is not always neurotic or self-defeating though. Moustakas (1972) contends that it is a necessary condition for individual growth. Constructive personal isolation results in the individual's knowing himself better through self-expression and self-renewal.

Personal isolation or loneliness has two distinct meanings. One is self-enhancing; the other is self-defeating. First, loneliness is the price one often pays for effective personal growth. Loneliness, or a sense of alienation, is experienced by the person when he rejects indiscriminate adherence to group demands which prevent him from establishing his own identity. Loneliness or personal isolation, in an existential sense, is an inescapable phenomenon that is necessary for personal growth. In man's existential loneliness or personal isolation, he finds time for reflection and thought because he is free from the distractions of his environment. Although there is psychological discomfort in loneliness or alienation, such feelings do not necessarily lend themselves to neurotic or self-defeating behavior if they are channeled in desired directions that lead to personal growth.

Personal isolation or loneliness, in a non-neurotic sense, is the result of a kind of existential nonconformity. An existential nonconformist is one who makes the most efficient use of his loneliness or personal isolation. He is a person who is self-assured, independent of external values, and can establish intimate contact with others readily (Tosi and Hoffman, 1972). Personal isolation or loneliness is not necessarily the antithesis of intimacy; surprisingly, it is involved in intimacy.

A second meaning of personal isolation or loneliness is neurotic or self-defeating. It is the result of one's lack of trust, industry, and personal identity. Neurotic isolation or loneliness in this sense is seen in a person's dire need to establish contact with others for the sake of countering his underlying feelings of rejection and inadequacy. The individual may avoid contact with others or else he may constantly want to be with others so that he has a feeling of intimacy. Although such pseudo-intimacy is not satisfying, he may be willing to settle for it and continue to experience self-defeating emotions.

Youth strive for interpersonal intimacy. For some — and perhaps too few — the striving is genuine. For the majority, the striving for interpersonal intimacy is complicated by dire needs for love, approval, belonging, and perfection. In short, the words and actions used to define and symbolize intimacy may be loaded with neurotic implications. Many of our youth, as well as adults, cannot discern effectively for themselves those meanings of intimacy which are self-enhancing from those which are self-defeating.

summary and conclusions

In summary, the developmental process from birth to adulthood has been described here. Attention was given to the development and the organization of the person or self. The self here was depicted as the cognitive, affective, and behavioral organization of the person's past experience and, to an extent, his future projections. It is the interplay of thinking, feelings, and behaving relative to one's situation or social environment and is responsible for the development of the self or of a person's personal belief and value system and behavioral orientation. Moreover, the interplay of self-processes suggests a unity or wholeness of the person operating within a socio-cultural system.

In conclusion, whether or not a person possesses a rational or self-enhancing philosophical belief system will depend largely on whether or not he has developed an adequate sense of basic trust, initiative, identity, and intimacy. Those of our youth who are dominated excessively by self-defeating emotions, such as mistrust, guilt, role-diffusion, and isolation, will need to learn new ways of overcoming these debilitating tendencies. For those of our youth whose self-development or personal growth has been stifled, certain experiences may be provided which are designed to facilitate personal growth. The counseling relationship offers a set of conditions whose aim is to facilitate the cognitive, the affective, and the behavioral development of the person towards the ultimate end of helping that person to realize, actualize, and affirm his potentialities. In the forthcoming sections, the counseling process, its stages, and requirements, and goals will be described.

stages of the counseling process

The process of counseling, psychotherapy, or any other helping relationship occurs within six general stages or levels. These stages are awareness, exploration, commitment, skill development, skill refinement, and, finally, change or redirection.* Each of these stages, while having its own separate characteristics, is contained in another, interacts with another, and influences another. For instance, when a person becomes more aware of his self-defeating thoughts, feelings, and behavior toward himself or another person, his awareness will increase as he explores and commits himself to change. Moreover, as he develops more effective personal and interpersonal skills, these new achievements will not only affect the level of his awareness, but will also be associated with a greater degree of exploration and commitment towards newer and more effective modes of living. The stages of the counseling process are in no way discrete entities. Each stage flows through the other (see Figure 3 on pages 14 and 15).

Most importantly, each of these stages should have its *counterpart* in the client's *real world*. When the client is helped by the counselor to become more aware of what is happening to him inside the counseling situation, he is also helped to become more aware of what is happening to him outside of the counseling situation. Such is the case for each stage. In other words, a major portion of the client's time is spent in the performing and practicing of appropriate behavioral modifying techniques outside of the counseling situation. Since there are about 112 hours per week during which the client is not in counseling, it seems only reasonable that a sufficient number of these hours be spent in more therapeutic ways of behaving.

A counselor needs to be sensitive or tuned into the particular level of client operation. He must be able to answer the following question

---

*These stages, identified by Quaranta (1971), have been adapted to counseling by the author.

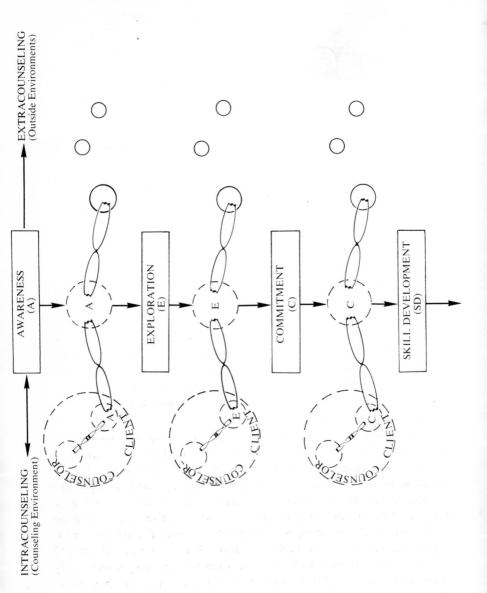

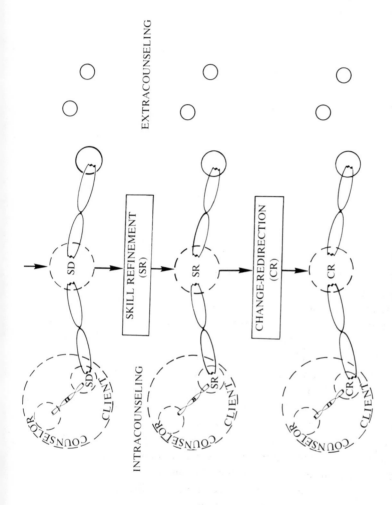

figure three

Stages of the Counseling Process*

*This illustration was developed by the author with special assistance from Dr. J. J. Quaranta.

15

with some degree of certainty. Relative to his problematic situation, is this client at an awareness level, an exploratory level, a commitment level, or at a skill development level? The answer to this question should dictate to some degree the nature of the intervention strategies employed by the counselors.

the awareness stage

In counseling or psychotherapy, it is crucial that the client become cognizant of the many new possibilities that the counseling process may offer him. Beyond the person's awareness of the need for help, it is important for him to realize that he may lack sufficient information and knowledge about effective living as well as the conditions under which to achieve a more effective life.

It is during this stage that the counselor actively introduces the client to the rudiments of the behavioral modifying process so that he may become better oriented to the demands of the counseling situation. Counselor-client roles and responsibilities should be discussed and the usual time limits established. Most importantly, however, the counselor and the client jointly should agree on both the short-term and the long-term goals to be achieved.

The counselor helps the client to become more aware of the counseling process within an interpersonal atmosphere of empathy, acceptance, and genuineness. Most importantly, the counselor communicates, through his words and actions, his expertise and competence. It is essential that the counselor be viewed and experienced by his client as an expert. As an expert, the counselor openly discusses with his client specific treatment interventions aimed at assisting the client in acquiring new modes of thinking about his problems.

As an adjunct to those processes occurring within the counseling situation, the counselor requires the client to initiate constructive action outside of the counseling relationship. At this awareness stage, outside activities might include reading books that describe the healthy personality and the counseling process itself.

The awareness stage of counseling primarily emphasizes the cognitive functioning of the client as the counselor directly assists the client in the acquisition of information and facts about the behavioral modifying process. As the client becomes more aware of the facts of counseling, he is able to explore himself more deeply with respect to his newly acquired information.

the exploration stage

The exploration stage involves the client's application of his newly acquired knowledge about effective living to himself. In other words, the client pursues the answer to the question of how this new information will affect his life. The counselor actively encourages the client to explore and translate these new inputs. This stage is a difficult one for the client. New modes of thinking, feeling, and behaving may contradict the client's already existing system of beliefs and values, and the client may experience excessive conflict or tension and show signs of strong resistance to the counseling process. But in spite of the client's resistance and uncertainty, the counselor actively and directly persists in his efforts to help the client explore himself more deeply. In a very calm, open, but sometimes forceful manner, the counselor demonstrates to his client the meaning of resistance and that while it is a naturally occurring phenomenon, it does inhibit the counseling process.

Initially, the exploration stage demands that the client cognitively explore more productive ways of behaving. Beyond a mere exposure to the benefits that may accrue as a result of counseling, the client must interpret or comprehend this new information and apply it to extra-counseling situations. When the client moves into the application phase of this stage, he is assisted by the counselor to appraise and to evaluate his new experience for the purpose of discovering new meanings in his life. Appraisal and evaluation are cognitive functions which are closely associated with one's basic belief and value system. When the client appraises and evaluates his situation relative to his internalized system of values, he moves into the affective or the emotional aspects of self.

The pragmatic application by the client of new self-knowledge to real world situations and his evaluation of the consequences of those new experiences may result in tendencies to approach or to avoid the emotional demands of the counseling process. It is at this point that some clients reject the counseling relationship and terminate it. Others may become defensive and resistant but remain willing to commit themselves to the counseling experience.

the commitment stage

With a greater awareness and exploration of self as he relates to the elements of the counseling process, the client, if he is to achieve more effective ways of living, must make a commitment to enter into a working alliance with the counselor. Commitment which grows out of personal knowledge serves as a source of his motivation for the client as he moves into the stage of skill development wherein he manifests or affirms that which he has explored. The commitment stage, while strongly affective in nature, is interwoven with the cognitive and affective properties of awareness and exploration.

Commitment, to a great extent, is based upon personalized knowledge but in another sense, it is sort of an act of faith (DeCharms, 1970). When the client enters into a working alliance with his counselor for the purpose of growing cognitively, emotionally, and behaviorally, he trusts that the counselor can indeed assist him in his growth. The counselor likewise commits himself to the client as a helper. The counselor also believes that his client is capable of developing many of the necessary skills for effective living — at least to some degree. Whatever goals were established jointly by the counselor and client, the counselor must be willing to commit himself to the client's attainment of his goals.

the skill development stage

Skill development is inherent in each stage of the counseling process. Up to this point, the client has acquired exploratory skills and skills relative to increased awareness of self and his situation. At this fourth stage of skill development, he must both learn and apply behavioral modifying procedures to his own self and his environment. In other words, as he acquires and learns new ways of thinking, feeling, and acting, he must practice them in real-life situations. At this stage, cognitive, affective, and behavioral processes must be given equal attention.

the skill refinement stage

The level of skill refinement is a logical progression from the preceding stage. The only difference at this level is that the client manifests or demonstrates more efficiently his newly acquired ways of thinking, feeling, and acting.

the change or redirection stage

The change or redirection stage implies that the client has become increasingly self-directed in assuming reponsibility for his behavior. There is evidence of substantial changes in his cognitive, affective, and behavioral-motoric processes. At this point, he appears to be a more effective person in one or maybe a variety of situations. If the counseling was of a type requiring minimum change and was limited to one specific client concern, it may be terminated at this point. If it is continued, the client recycles or redirects himself through the six stages of the counseling process. This second recycling may be accomplished with less difficulty, although this may not always be the case.

aims of counseling: personal growth

The counseling process is designed to facilitate and to enhance the personal-social growth of the individual and is directed towards some set of goals which may be immediate or long-range. Ultimately and ideally, it would be desirable for persons involved in the counseling process to reach a high level of personal functioning or self-realization. Immediately and practically, however, it is important that persons successively approximate ultimately higher levels of functioning. In 1965, E. L. Shostrom addressed the question of the goals and processes of personal growth in counseling and psychotherapy. He devised an instrument, the Personal Orientation Inventory (1965), as a way of assessing one's personal gains as a result of counseling and psychotherapy. The dimensions of personal growth or self-realization developed by Shostrom which can easily be translated into counseling goals include the following aspects:

Time Competence refers to one's ability to live his life in the "here and now"—a present orientation as opposed to a past or future orientation. Time competence also implies a balance between the immediate gratification of one's desires, wishes, or needs and being able to delay gratification for the sake of long-term rewards and satisfaction. Time competence suggests the delicate balance between "long-term" and "short-term" hedonism.

Inner-Directedness is the ability to be positively self-oriented and self-directed in contradiction to being directed by others. Inner-directedness implies the capacity of a person to think for himself instead of having others think for him.

Existentiality is the ability of a person to react to new experiences without rigid adherence to unsound, unscientific, or unproven principles. Existentiality has to do with an openness to experience or one's ability to approach new experiences without making premature, biased, and prejudiced judgments.

Feeling Reactivity refers to one's awareness and sensitivity to his thoughts, feelings, and desires. It is an "in-tuneness" with self.

Spontaneity is the freedom to react or act in a nondefensive, reasonable manner in a variety of interpersonal situations. It suggests an affirmation of one's self within social arenas.

Self-Regard is a dimension of personal growth that is almost synonomous with self-respect. It refers to a person's being able to affirm himself because of his self-defined sense of worth or value to himself.

Self-Acceptance refers to one's ability to accept himself fully in spite of his biological, sociological, and psychological limitations. The person unconditionally accepts his own fallibility and the fact that others might see him as a fallible person. Moreover, self-acceptance is the intrapersonal basis for accepting others and their fallibility. Self-acceptance implies that one does not ascribe such evaluative labels as "good" and "bad" to total sense of self. One's performances may be evaluated, but they are not to be confused with "total selfhood."

Nature of Man as an aspect of growth depicts one's affirming a rational-realistic, constructive view of man. As a philosophical orientation, it is opposed to the more unsound, unproven, dogmatic, and magical-mystical philosophical positions.

Synergy is a cognitive ability which allows a person to seek higher-level solutions to problematic situations; in other words, it is the ability to transcend seemingly opposite positions or to synthesize them into a meaningful concept. Synergy also suggests creative thoughts.

Acceptance of Aggression is the capacity to accept one's natural aggressiveness as opposed to defensiveness, denial, and repression of aggression.

Capacity for Intimate Contact is the facility to develop close interpersonal relationships with others unencumbered by expectations and obligations.

Personal growth refers to growth in all of the above areas. We can think of short-term and long-term growth as being a result of counseling in terms of the degree to which a person progresses or develops along these twelve dimensions in a given time frame.

In a recent study, Tosi and Hoffman (1972) submitted the Personal Orientation Inventory to a factor analysis, a statistical technique which examines the interrelationships between the subscales of a particular test and reduces the number of subscales to a few which are called factors. Specifically, the scales of the Personal Orientation Inventory were reduced to three factors—open-mindedness, existential non-conformity, and extraversion. A general interpretation would suggest that the scale describes the healthy or reasonable person as one who is open to experience, can function independently but still relates effectively to others, and can affirm himself through independent action.

summary

Several parameters of human growth and development were explored in this chapter. A model or conceptual scheme was provided which served as a guide to the fundamental social-psychological processes associated with personal development. Personal growth from infancy to adulthood was then described along with the many conditions which inhibit as well as facilitate it.

The counseling process, as one alternative way of intervening in the personal development of persons—and youth in particular—was described in terms of several stages—awareness, exploration, commitment, skill development, skill refinement, and change and redirection. Finally, the aim or goal of counseling, self-realization or self-actualization, was described in terms of twelve dimensions.

In Chapter Two, we will move from a global consideration of the human condition and of intervention to many specific ideas and concepts about emotional disturbance and counseling. Chapter 2 introduces the basic philosophy and concepts of rational-emotive theory and counseling—a method of intervention which I believe to be one of the most sensible, realistic, and effective means of helping individuals grow in very personal ways. As we shall see, it is a didactic-experiential-directive method of counseling.

two * rational-emotive counseling: philosophy and concepts

Rational-emotive counseling, as does any system of counseling, consists of a philosophy of man which is related to the practice of it. This chapter explicates most of the central philosophical and conceptual themes contained in rational-emotive theory and practice.

Viewing as it does man's nature as being neither essentially good nor essentially evil and assuming the position that man defines or creates himself or his essence, rational-emotive (RE) counseling is an attempt to teach a person to acquire the skill required to become his own therapist so he can take charge of himself and facilitate his own growth. To accomplish this, the RE counselor needs to provide his client with an atmosphere which maximizes such an outcome. For instance, RE theory suggests the importance of the counselor's ability to be genuine, empathic, and unconditional in his regard for the client. The theory also suggests that the RE counselor actively and directly combat his clients' emotional disturbances through confrontation, teaching, and re-education.

The following topics are discussed in this chapter from a rational-emotive point of view: personal worth, emotional disturbance, confrontation, persuasion and influence, criteria for rational thinking, insight and self-understanding, and the facilitative or relationship conditions (empathy, respect, concreteness, immediacy, genuineness, self-disclosure, psychological teaching and re-education, and homework).

personal worth and self-acceptance

Most systems or theories of counseling and psychotherapy are based upon assumptions regarding man's essential nature. Some philosophers and behavioral scientists have turned towards theoretical or metaphysical explanations of man which go beyond that which can be observed or is readily apparent, while other philosophers and scientists rely on their observations and the results of empirical research in order to build a model of man. Both the deductive and inductive methods of inquiry are facts which cannot be denied and probably are both quite necessary in obtaining knowledge.

In spite of our methods of inquiry—whether they be experimental-inductive, nonexperimental-deductive, or simply descriptive—we do make assumptions about man's nature. In the field of counseling, there are those who view man's essential nature as being evil and who therefore go from there to counteract this evil with their therapeutic interventions. Others, for the most part humanists, assume that man is by nature good and if he becomes evil or wicked, it is because of other influences. For instance, certain Judeo-Christian existentialists believe that man's nature is inherently good just because he exists. Other existential thinkers and some radical empiricists disagree with this assumption and hold that man by nature is neither good nor evil. For the radical empiricists, the question can only be answered through experimental means. Existentialists, without denying the experimental and scientific method, also greatly emphasize man's subjective experiencing and his ability to define himself as a valid source of knowledge. Existential thinkers who refuse to make assumptions about man's inherent good or evil are willing to assert that man creates his own essence, or that which he is, through his own choices and actions. Moreover, these existentialists emphasize man's being and becoming rather than his innate worth or worthlessness, goodness or badness as the most crucial elements to his existence.

In agreement with certain existentialists, such as Sartre (1956), rational-emotive theory emphasizes man's unique ability to determine for himself that which he can be or become in spite of the many biological, sociological, political, economical, and psychological constraints which mitigate against this. On the matter of man's intrinsic worth or worthlessness, Ellis (1962) asserts that such notions are definitional. Furthermore, such definitions may be ascribed to one by others and therefore be extrinsic or they can be self-ascribed and therefore intrinsic. Since these notions are not statements of fact, they cannot be proven or disproven. Moreover, there is danger of striving needlessly and compulsively to define oneself as worthwhile in order to avoid the other half of the definition—worthlessness. Rational-emotive theory deemphasizes concepts such as personal worth and worthlessness and stresses man's becoming a more efficient and a happier person. That is, RE counselors help their clients develop a willingness to spend most of their lives discovering what they want to do and actively doing that which they want to do rather than accepting extrinsic values placed upon them by others as having intrinsic value; a greater commitment to the process of life rather than to ultimate goals or ends (Simply stated, this involves "living in the here and now" without losing sight of some long-range goals.); and an acceptance of self as doer or creative person rather than as passive receiver who is totally dependent upon others. The client's worth or value has meaning when it is personal and is largely an outgrowth of constructive actions. Even then, its meaning is somewhat vague, and if it is to make any sense at all, such definitions should be related to the person's own being and becoming (Ellis, 1962).

Ellis has engaged the objectivist psychologist Nathaniel Branden in a debate on the matter of self-esteem and self-worth. Branden (1967) points out that self-esteem is a belief or conviction that one is competent to live and worthy of living. Branden's assertion that human beings tend to define themselves as worthless if they are incompetent, stupid, neurotic, or psychotic leads to a conclusion which implies that one would have low-self esteem if he were stupid, incompetent, or insane, since these faults would be a reflection of his inability to deal with reality. Although Ellis (1968) agrees with Branden, he takes exception to Branden's conclusions, places conditions of worth within the individual himself, and simply deemphasizes external conditions of worth. He contends that it is possible for a person to acknowledge that he may indeed be more incompetent, stupid, or psychotic than others but *accept* fully the fact that he is of *value to himself*.[1] If a person accepts the notion that he is human, alive, and deserves to exist and be personally happy, he will pose conditions which largely contradict any ideas that suggest that he is totally worthless.

[1]Self-acceptance in rational-emotive theory is perhaps its most important concept. This idea implies that a person is of value to himself because he exists and is alive as a human being. The assumption is made that existence and aliveness are better than being dead—for if one exists, it is possible for one to create himself. If he is dead, the possibility for humanly creating himself does not exist. Self-acceptance means that one does not evaluate his total being in terms of his performances — whether they are to his liking or to his disliking. Since man is by definition fallible, it would be in his best interest to accept his fallibility and to try to improve on his strengths as well as his weaknesses. If he is successful — fine. If he fails — tough. Whether he succeeds or fails, he still has his existence and aliveness.

emotional disturbance

Emotional disturbances are usually experienced by people in the form of excessive states of anxiety, worry or fear, boredom, failure to achieve, anger and hostility, frustration, guilt or self-condemnation, depression, loneliness, self-pity, uncontrolability, and inferiority. Such emotional states, when intense, are associated with a variety of self-defeating actions or behaviors. Among these undesirable behavioral manifestations are tardiness, avoidance of responsibilities and situations, lack of self-discipline, demanding approval and attention. Rational-emotive therapy postulates that one's emotions are primarily a function of one's thinking; since emotions and thinking overlap significantly, they are virtually the same process (Ellis, 1962).

Arnold (1960) hypothesizes that emotions are simply the evaluations or appraisals a person ascribes to a given phenomenon which have a strong affective or bodily component. Evaluation, which is essentially a cognitive function, involves both perceiving and responding. Furthermore, emotions and values seem to be the premise-based conclusions a person has accepted about a given thing (Branden, 1962).

Ellis asserts that:

> A good deal—though not necessarily all—of what we call emotion, therefore, would seem to be a kind of appraisal or thinking that (a) is strongly slanted or biased by previous perceptions or experiences; that (b) is highly personalized; that, (c) is often accompanied by gross bodily reactions; and (d) that it is likely to induce the emoting individual to take some kind of positive or negative action. What we usually call thinking would seem to be a more tranquil, less personalized, less systematically involved for, at least perceived, and less activity-directed mode of discriminating.[2]

He further states that:

> In any event, assuming that you don't at the very beginning have any conscious or unconscious thoughts accompanying your emotion, it appears to be almost impossible to sustain an emotional outburst without bolstering it by repeated ideas. For unless you keep telling yourself something on the order of "Oh, my heavens! How terrible it would have been if that car had hit me!" your fright over almost being hit by the car will soon die. And unless you keep telling yourself, when you are punched on the jaw by someone, "that fellow

[2]A. Ellis, *Reason and Emotion in Psychotherapy* (New York: Lyle Stuart, 1962), p. 48. Copyright © 1962 by the Institute for Rational Living, Inc. Published by arrangement with Lyle Stuart, Inc.

who punched me on the jaw is a villain! I hope he gets his just desserts!" the pain of being punched will soon die and your anger at this fellow will die with the pain.[3]

Much of that which we call emotion is nothing more than internalized words, sentences, or phrases. Oftentimes, certain signs or symbols may be associated with strong negative or positive affects, but even in those cases, such signs and symbols can be reduced to prejudiced, biased, or evaluative words, phrases, or sentences. Moreover, most sustained negative emotions are, according to Ellis:

> . . . the result of stupidity, ignorance, or disturbances, and for the most part they may be, and should be, eliminated by the application of knowledge and straight thinking. For if perpetuated states of emotion generally follow from the individual's conscious or unconscious thinking: and if his thinking is, in turn, mainly a concommitant to his self-verbalization, then it would follow that he is rarely affected (made sad or glad) by outside things and events: rather he is affected by his perceptions, attitudes, or internalized sentences about outside things and events.[4]

Emotional disturbances within the rational-emotive framework are, in large measure, functions of cognitive or thought processes, especially those which are evaluative in nature. Negative affective states and their behavioral manifestations are, in most instances, caused and maintained by biased, prejudiced, and illogical evalutive thinking. Moreover, such thoughts generally are associated with belief and attitudinal systems.

Technically, Lindsley (1957) has observed that present perceptual discriminations or past perceptual discriminations stored as memories, the ideas and images, and the higher-level symbolic and thought processes in the human organism are quite capable of generating impulses in the cortex regions of the brain. Such impulses excite the reticular formation which then induces electrocortical changes in the direction of activation in the organism. Emotion is conceived as the arousal of various, activating patterns which involve a highly complex neural mechanism.

Many complex factors are associated with emotional phenomena. At least three major origins or pathways of emotion have been identified. These are sensori-motor processes, biophysical stimulation, and biophysical stimulation through the cognitive, symbolic thinking process (Ellis, 1962).

[3]*Ibid.*, p. 49.
[4]*Ibid.*, p. 58.

In counseling and psychotherapy, the task of the counselor or therapist is to help his client become aware of the basis for his emotional disturbance; to help him explore new ways of thinking and to contradict those illogical, self-defeating, or neurotic thoughts; to persuade the client to commit himself to his own personal growth; and to teach or help the client gain for himself those skills necessary for him to become a more effective person.

confrontation

Rational-emotive counseling makes a systematic and intensive use of confrontation. The rational-emotive counselor wastes little or no time in getting to the client's core concerns. Regardless of the client's expressed content about a problematic situation, the counselor focuses his direct attention on the client's internalized philosophic beliefs about those situations. To express this somewhat differently, we can say that the counselor enters the client's system of personal and internalized meanings associated with his experiences. Since internalized meanings often are not manifested readily by the client and exist or operate at a latent level, and because, moreover, persons easily distort their own meanings (Kemp, 1961; Tosi, 1970), the counselor's task of bringing the client's symbolized experiences into awareness is an arduous one.

Initially, resistance from the client is obvious and to be expected as a response to counselor confrontation, but this is quite normal and understandable behavior. Why shouldn't a person resist even when some dedicated and interested person takes the time, the energy, and the patience to challenge and to attack the irrational thinking and ideas or philosophies that are at the core of his emotional-behavioral disturbances? When the client has been indoctrinated and taught to think and believe about himself in highly self-defeating ways, the counselor should not only fully expect that he will encounter stubbornness and resistance but he should also find it obvious and accept unconditionally the client's hesitancy to commit himself to the counseling process. But since openness to experience, in contrast to obstinate and irrational resisting, is central to the client's effective functioning, the counselor proceeds to confront forcefully his client's inconsistencies in his believing and thinking. As an outgrowth of the confrontation, the counselor must then proceed actively and directly to help the client to reconstruct his belief system.

In particular, rational-emotive counselors employ the *ABCD* method of problem analysis and confrontation. This method provides the client with a cognitive framework from which much of his thinking, emoting, and behaving relative to most problematic situations can be clearly understood. In a very direct, persuasive, and sometimes forceful manner, the counselor helps the client to analyze his problematic situation or the internal-external events (A) about which the client became upset. He then determines, through verbal and nonverbal cues given by the client, what the client is telling himself (B) about (A) (an activating event). If the client is emotionally disturbed, he is usually telling himself at (B) something illogical, absurd, or stupid about (A); this is the cause of his emotional disturbance (C). (D) designates the behavioral manifestation of (B) and (C). (B) can be reduced to a set of irrational sentences or beliefs (IBs) and a set of more reasonable or sane beliefs (RBs). The counselor merely helps the client to become aware of and explore both sets of beliefs and helps him to commit himself to more reasonable ways through teaching, persuading, illustrating, and reindoctrinating. Conditions are arranged by the counselor and the client both inside and outside of the one-to-one relationship for the client to experience and later acquire the skills for becoming a more effective person.

Before the client moves exclusively into skill development, he must become aware of and explore, inside and outside of the counseling situation, those sets of (RBs) which are in contradiction with his (IBs). This awareness and exploration are facilitated and expedited when the counselor is active in explicating these through the ABCD paradigm. The rule is one of confronting the client's (IBs), challenging them, contradicting them, and ultimately replacing them with (RBs). It should be kept in mind that negative emotions and irrational thinking and believing are virtually one and the same process. Positive emotions, on the other hand, are associated with more rational ways of thinking and believing.

In rational-emotive counseling, confrontation is a frequent occurrence, especially during the stages of awareness, exploration, and commitment. When the client enters the skill development and skill refinement stages, there are rather obvious signs that he is taking charge of his own self-development. At these latter two stages, the frequency and intensity of the counselor's active-directive confrontations are decreased. It is as if the client is becoming his own counselor.

persuasion and influence

The counselor's influence and persuasive abilities are associated with changes in client attitudes and belief systems. Factors related to the influence process are the counselor's expertise and his trustworthiness.

Counseling effectiveness is enhanced when the client perceives the counselor as an expert. Moreover, there is increasing evidence that the explicit structuring of the counseling process by the counselor affects the client's perceptions of the counselor's expertise (Truax, 1966) as well as enhancing the counselor's image as an influence agent. When the counselor is able to provide the client with a sensible framework in which to view his problematic situations and can explicate the specific elements within that framework (i.e., problem-solving stategies, goals, and objectives), it is much easier for the client to engage in constructive action, since he does not have to waste needless time entertaining and making sense out of a possibly ambiguous situation.

In his book *Persuasion and Healing*, Jerome Frank (1963) recognizes the importance of the counselor's persuasive potency. More recently, Truax has found that counselors who are more persuasive are more effective with their clients than those counselors who are less persuasive. Truax, however, has not been too explicit as to the meaning of persuasion, while Frank, in part, has attached a magical meaning to persuasion by pointing out the similarities between the witch doctor who exorcises evil spirits from possessed persons and psychotherapists who combat mental disturbances.

In rational-emotive theory, persuasion has an explicit meaning. It is the counselor's persistent demonstrating and illustrating to the client of how his irrational thoughts and beliefs are associated with or, for the most part, the cause of his emotional-behavioral disorders. In rational-emotive counseling, persuasion is not rooted in magic or mysticism but in reason and experimentation. The counselor uses reason and logic, empirical evidence, and the client's personal-experiential testing of hypotheses as the foundation of persuasion. Moreover, if the client does ascribe magical powers and attributes to the counselor, the counselor wastes no time in challenging such meanings and pointing out their self-defeating nature.

Magical and mystical persuasion has no place in rational-emotive counseling. There is reason to believe that symptom reduction in neurotic persons may be a function of general placebo reactivity or of one's expectations that a therapist has the power to cure (even though there is no therapeutic intervention). Under such conditions, however, reduction in symptoms may not reflect substantive changes in client functioning. As a matter of fact, symptom reduction of this sort may simply reinforce in the client his already pernicious beliefs about magic and healing. Changes in client expectations and belief play an important role in allaying neurotic disturbances when the change is in a direction of reason. One major goal of RE counseling is to help the client acquire a set of rational-realistic-constructive beliefs or expectations about himself, the counselor's professional strengths and limitations, and the world as a whole.

The persuasive ability of the counselor and the extent to which he can be a positive influence on his client are ultimately functions of his expertise as an agent for behavioral change and his ability to communicate his expertise to his client via his own commitment to the personal growth and development of that client. The commitment generally will be perceived and experienced by the client. Even though the client may resist and at times go so far as to deny his own therapeutic progress, he later will perceive or believe that the counselor is acting in his (the client's) best interest.

If one equates the persuasive ability of the effective counselor with the persuasive ability of the dishonest used car dealer, he is mistaken. The dishonest car salesman may sell a faulty car, but the lie is soon discovered by the buyer and, in time, the dealer's credibility is lost. The committed counselor actively and directively uses his art of persuasion to induce the client to challenge his own self-defeating emotions and to become a more reasonable, happy, efficient, freedom-aspiring, responsible human being.

Persuasion in rational-emotive counseling is not to be confused with the practices of some of our contemporary faith healers and evangelists who try to induce persons to place their total lives in the hands of Jesus Christ or any other deity. Rational-emotive counselors denounce unquestioned adherence to supernatural forces who supposedly govern our lives. Moreover, they question and challenge many of the ideas of such recent trends as the Jesus Movement in which followers try to convince themselves and others that one can only be saved or happy if one gives his life up for Jesus. Rational-emotive counselors work diligently to persuade their more religious-minded clients that they would be better to accept the philosophy, "The Lord helps those who help themselves." To reiterate: Persuasion in rational-emotive counseling is inextricably interwoven with reason, logic, and personal hypotheses-testing. Mysticism, cultism, magic, and witchcraft are rejected and have no real place in the RE system.

insight and self-understanding

RE counseling emphasizes three forms of insight and/or self-understanding. The first insight consists of the client's realization that his present behavior is, to a great extent, a function of antecedent conditions. But, more importantly, the antecedents of the client's emotional disturbance exist in the present and take the form of irrational ideas or nonsensical self-definition. A second type of insight involves the awareness and understanding of how the client organizes, perpetuates, and sustains his early adopted destructive philosophies and ideas. That is, he discovers how he maintains his own self-indoctrinations, even though he may have originally learned these tendencies from significant others. The third insight has to do with the awareness and acceptance that the client can greatly promote his personal growth through hard work and practice. Most importantly, the emotionally upset client must learn to attack vigorously his irrational ideas and behavior in spite of the many biological and sociological factors working against him. In short, the client needs to affirm his new self-understandings and acceptance in both thought and constructive action.

In summary, we can say that the RE counselor actively aids his client in the attainment of greater awareness or self-insights in three ways. In addition, he proceeds by helping the client accept for himself these insights. And, finally, he stresses that this client affirms these insights in the form of a self-enhancing philosophy and in reasonable and constructive actions.

criteria for rational thinking

RE counseling is a re-educative experience for a person in which the counseling process ultimately is aimed at the attainment of higher levels of self-realization. But in order for a person to become a more actualized person, he must learn the characteristics of rational thinking. Thinking is rational when it meets the folowing three criteria (Maultsby, 1970): it leads to constructive actions that are likely to preserve the individual's life; it stimulates actions that have a greater likelihood of achieving the individual's personally defined goals; and it does not result in significant and sustained personal, emotional, or environmental conflict (*significant* here refers to amounts not calmly accepted by the person). If a person's thinking does not meet these three criteria, the chances are it is not rational. RE counselors teach their clients to pose their thinking against these criteria both inside and outside of the counseling relationship until rational thought patterns become consistent.

Rational or critical thinking about oneself is among the most significant factors contributing to one's growth and development (Guilford, 1967; Kemp, 1961; Maslow, 1962; Rokeach, 1961; Tosi and Hoffman, 1972). It should be kept in mind that when a person engages in higher-order rational thinking about himself, it does not necessarily mean that he will arrive at one and only one conclusion or solution to his problem (convergent thought production); he may arrive at several conclusions or solutions that fit the above three criteria (divergent thought production).

the facilitative conditions in rec

In a number of theoretical and research papers Carl Rogers (1958, 1962) has identified several necessary and sufficient conditions for counseling and psychotherapy practices. These conditions, all of which are counselor or therapist-expressed attitudes, consist of empathy, congruence, unconditional positive regard, and level of regard. Rogers has hypothesized that when counselors or therapists offer their clients high levels of these conditions, results are more positive than when low levels of these conditions are offered.

More recently, Roger's position has been extended and modified by several contemporary psychologists (Alexik and Carkhuff, 1967; Cannon and Carkhuff, 1969; Carkhuff, 1969, 1972; Truax, 1966, VanderVeen 1961). Specifically, Carkhuff (1969) has extended Roger's conditions for effective counseling and placed them under the rubric of "facilitative" rather than "necessary and sufficient." The "facilitative conditions," as identified by Carkhuff, consist of accurate empathy, respect, concreteness, immediacy, confrontation, genuineness, and self-disclosure.

There is reason to believe (Tosi, 1970; Tosi, 1973) that when counselors are rational, they are perceived by their clients as offering higher levels of these facilitative or attitudinal conditions than do those counselors who are less rational. Correspondingly, when clients hold more reasonable belief systems, they are more likely to perceive the counselors as offering these facilitative conditions. RE counselors believe in the importance of these "process" or "facilitative" conditions in the counseling relationship but do make some modification in them and add some conditions of their own. For instance, teaching, re-evaluation, and outside counseling homework assignments often are considered facilitative conditions by RE counselors.

accurate empathy

Accurate empathy refers to the counselor's ability to respond to the client's thoughts, feelings, and behavior with understanding. The counselor must be able to communicate his full awareness and understanding of his client's underlying concerns. Accurate empathy and its expression by the counselor are related to the client's depth of self-exploration.

respect

The counselor manifests respect for his client when he demonstrates that he is committed to the client's growth and development. In rational-emotive counseling and psychotherapy, the counselor gives evidence of this trait by a high degree of activity and involvement in the counseling process.

concreteness

Concreteness is synonomous with specificity. The counselor involves and guides the client in the expression of specific thoughts, feelings, and behaviors. Although an RE counselor ultimately strives to help a person develop a meaningful and rational philosophy of life, he first attends to his client's more specific concerns, thereby enabling the client to focus and attend to specific aspects of a more global orientation towards life.

immediacy

Immediacy refers to the counselor's translation of the client's insights and understandings to terms of the counselor-client relationship in the here and now. The counselor encourages the client to express his thoughts, feelings, and behaviors towards him; in psychoanalytical terms, he focuses upon the attitudes and feelings the client projects onto him. The counselor confronts these projections and demonstrates their appropriateness or inappropriateness in the present relationship. The rational-emotive counselor is also quick to point out the client's irrational projections and proclivities outside of the counseling relationship.

In RE counseling, immediacy is an important variable, but it does not necessarily outweigh the necessity of bridging the gap between the client's experiencing and learning inside the counseling relationship and in the outside world. Moreover, RE counselors do not become compulsive about the here and now. After all, the client lives most of his life outside of the counseling situation. It is all too easy for some clients to become overly concerned with the here and now only to forget the meaningful considerations of future possibilities. Or they use the jargon of the here and now as an excuse for their self-defeating behavior.

genuineness

The facilitative condition of genuineness refers to the counselor's open-mindedness and authenticity as a person. The counselor's genuineness or openness is affirmed in his natural, spontaneous, and nondefensive responses to his client. In RE counseling, genuineness is manifested by the counselor's fearless attempts to intervene directly and sometimes forcefully in the life of the client. When the counselor manifests such an attitudinal condition, he also serves as a healthy model for the client.

Many investigations have shown that counselors who are open-minded or genuine are better able to establish a working alliance with their clients (Allen, 1967; Carkhuff, 1969; Tosi, 1970). It appears that when counselors and psychotherapists have open or reasonable belief systems, they are better able to empathize with their clients and much more tolerant of individual client differences; hence, they have a greater tendency to approach the counseling relationship with less anxiety (Kemp 1961; Tosi 1970).

self-disclosure

Self-disclosure is the willingness of the counselor to reveal significant aspects of his own personal development. It is used widely as a technique or a condition of the counseling relationship by some existential relationship-oriented counselors. Moreover, Jourard (1971) has presented rather convincing evidence that client self-disclosure is facilitated when the counselor discloses something of himself.

It is true that virtually all counselors and psychotherapists prefer that their clients disclose significant areas of their lives. There are also instances when it is appropriate for a counselor to disclose himself as a means of encouraging a greater openness on the client's part. But many successful Freudian, Adlerian, and behavioral counselors do not make a habit of disclosing themselves. As a matter of fact, for them, therapist self-disclosure is an irrelevant condition.

RE counselors reveal aspects of their own lives only when it is appropriate for them to do so. Unlike some of our contemporary humanistic expressive-emotive counselors, they do not disclose themselves to their clients unwittingly, needlessly, and indiscriminately. As an instance of a case where self-disclosure would be appropriate, we might say that, to demonstrate his own fallibility to a client, an RE counselor might select some instance from his life whereby he overcame and conquered some emotional disturbance.

psychological teaching and re-education

One of the major activities of the RE counselor is teaching, for the counselor teaches the client who suffers from emotional disturbance to question, to challenge, and to expel his unscientific hypothesis or beliefs about himself. Ellis (1970) has asserted that:

> We teach, and the main thing we teach is scientific methods, just as a physics teacher or a psychology teacher, especially an experimental psychology teacher, teaches his students. Lots of people who

have never had any real contact with scientific thinking unconsciously, unwittingly use it. But many others mainly think unscien-
tifically. We show these individuals that when they are no damned
good, this is a hypothesis, and we teach them to ask themselves,
"Where is the evidence to sustain this hypothesis?" In science, you
set up a hypothesis, and you try to find confirmatory or noncon-
firmatory evidence."[5]

The key assumption or value here is that scientific thinking about
oneself is more productive than is magical thinking or simple blind,
unscientific thinking. The RE counselor spends a great deal of time
re-educating his clients. Specifically, he teaches his client in an authoritative manner (as opposed to an authoritarian manner) how to think for
himself.

For the RE counselor, the teaching-educating-reconstructing dimension of the counseling process is a facilitative condition. The didactic
experiential approach in REC is essential because it is the obvious step
beyond empathy, respect, and acceptance. Therefore, if there are necessary conditions for a rational-emotive counseling relationship, teaching
and re-education should be included among these.

One should not conclude erroneously that RE counselors are
pedantic authoritarians who theorize and lecture their clients without regard for their personhood. On the contrary, RE counselors are in the
serious business of cognitive, emotional, and behavioral re-education.
When we teach a person to challenge and to reconstruct his previous
ways of thinking and acting, it is requisite that we do understand and
accept his feelings — be tuned in to his feelings. Since a person's internalized beliefs occur in the form of thoughts, sentences, or symbols which
are closely associated with his affective or feeling states, they are virtually
one and the same phenomenon; when RE counselors encounter the recal-
citrant patterns of their client's emotional disturbances through cognitive
thought processes, their directive and active teachings are indeed appropriate and necessary if such ingrained cognitive, affective, and behavioral systems are to be modified substantially.

homework

The use of systematic homework, or extra-counseling assignments, is
an important and essential adjunct to the learning which occurs during
the counseling session, since counseling is more effective when it
emphasizes the acquisition of new and more constructive behaviors in

[5]A. Ellis, "A Humanistic Approach to Psychotherapy," *The Humanist* (1970):
50-51.

a variety of extra-counseling situations (Goldstein, Heller, Sechrest, 1966.) Moreover, the efficacy of counseling is increased when arrangements are made to provide the client with the means of conceptualizing new experiences during as well as outside the counseling sessions. In other words, learning will be facilitated when the client develops a cognitive structure to use in anticipating, organizing, and understanding new and more self-enhancing ways of feeling and behaving (Ausubel, 1960; Goldstein, Heller, Sechrest, 1966; Kelly, 1955).

Interestingly, rational-emotive counseling provides the client with a cognitive basis from which his new thoughts, feelings, and actions can be viewed in a more meaningful and constructive manner. The ABC method of analysis of problems and emotional disturbances is an example of the use of this base. The ABC method provides the client with a global or more inclusive theory of his own behavior; through it, the client is more aware of the behavior of others and able to interpret and understand that behavior more easily.

Use of the "in vivo" techniques is a strategy which translates a counseling theory into a real-life experience for a client. RE counselors insist that their clients adopt a pragmatic experimental philosophy by submitting their beliefs and ideas about life to reality testing. In addition, RE counselors influence and instruct their clients within the counseling situation, although if the client is to make a substantive personal progress, it is he who must practice his newly discovered ideas and behavior outside of the counseling situation. It is almost exclusively through outside effort and work on the client's part that real and long-lasting changes occur. RE counselors strive to provide conditions inside and outside the counseling situation which facilitate the client's personal development and self-realization.*

---

*It should be noted that although confrontation is listed as one of the facilitative conditions by Carkhuff. It is not included in this discussion since it has been described earlier in RE terms.

three * the irrational ideas

Rational-emotive theory is built upon a foundation which emphasizes the development of the person within a socio-cultural system. The theory, being a humanistic one, emphasizes cogently the process through which an individual organizes and develops a personal philosophy or orientation towards life. Fundamentally, this personal philosophy is one's internalized system of values and beliefs or meanings and the affirming of these in the world. When persons become emotionally disturbed, their disturbances are observed not only in faulty behavior patterns but also in concomitant irrational thought patterns. Rational-emotive theory holds that while emotional disturbance and biased, prejudiced thinking and believing are virtually one in the same thing, it is one's irrational thinking and believing that serves to elicit, perpetuate, and sustain emotional disturbance.

The process of personal growth or self-realization demands, almost by definition, that a person be able to reflect upon his existence, assess his being, expand his awareness of self, explore himself and his relationship to the world, and make the personal commitments necessary to gain the competencies required to construct and affirm a reasonable and self-enhancing philosophy of life; therefore, a person will need to recognize, contradict, challenge, and reconstruct at a higher level those personal beliefs and values that inhibit his growth.

Ellis (1961) has identified a set of irrational ideas or beliefs which are commonly espoused by most persons and which are particularly noticeable in our youth. Resulting from indoctrination by parents, significant others, and the various media, these ideas and beliefs and a person's unquestioning loyalty and adherence to them are associated with several pernicious emotional states, including guilt, shame, depression, and anxiety. Ellis's irrational ideas as they apply to youth make up the major focus of this chapter. These irrational ideas, their negative emotional consequences, and their rational alternatives are explored in this chapter.

Irrational Idea One: All persons have an absolute need for love and approval from most of their peers and other significant persons, such as parents and teachers.

This pernicious belief probably is rooted in the child's early interaction with his parents. If the child's parents are not personally confident and secure, they no doubt communicate such an attitude to the child. Any lack of trust or security in self is often associated with anxiety and can lead one to seek out security in others; if a person is successful in gaining the love and the approval of others (a sense of security in others), he is quite likely to feel less anxious. But the temporary reduction of anxiety resulting from the immediate gratification of one's needs for love and approval may not always be in the individual's best interest for this anxiety reduction is likely to reinforce one's belief that he must be loved and approved by virtually everyone in order to feel worthwhile as a person.

In the temporary absence of love and approval, a person becomes even more anxious or depressed if he convinces himself that he must have these needs fulfilled if he is to survive. Unless the person eventually concludes that total approval and love from most significant others is unnecessary, he will experience much unhappiness in his life. If one concludes more sensibly that his sense of personal worth is self-defined and that it does not have to be defined for him by others he will be better off. While it is desirable to be approved and loved by others, one does not have to sacrifice his own sense of identity to achieve this state. Just because young children require love and approval from significant persons, it does not mean adults require it in the same way. One should strive to be approved and loved if he wants to, but if he is not successful to the degree he might like, he does not have to become needlessly upset or convince himself that he is a "louse." Just because one lacks love and approval at any given moment does not mean that he will never have them in the future. The tendency, however, for most people is to convince themselves that if they don't have love and approval now, they never will and that they can't possibly survive alone.

Recently, several graduate students criticized me and another professor for not practicing some of the things counselors supposedly preach—namely, close, warm, and empathetic interpersonal caring or relating. The criticism went something like this: "You professors only care about yourselves and your publications and outside consultations. We need you to relate to us personally. You should care for us and attend to our needs and wants. Your behavior makes us angry and depressed. We want and demand that you relate to us in more humanistic ways." It was true that most of the professors on our counseling staff had not been attending to the students in the most desirable ways educationally—not because we all are totally selfish "ego maniacs" but because we were operating with about half of the number of staff necessary to run large Ph.D. and Master's degree programs in addition to some new undergraduate programs in education. Even so, the students' observations were generally correct. It was their interpretation of the facts that was somewhat distorted; more specifically, it was their own neurotic demands that they should be loved, approved, and totally attended to by us that were irrational. When we finally entered into a dialogue with them, we confronted and supported their reasonable demands but also showed them how they were disturbing themselves needlessly because they were not achieving what they wanted.

Many professors and teachers also believe that they must be loved and approved by virtually all of their students if they are to be considered effective and worthwhile teachers. I personally believe that this is nonsense. While I do prefer to be liked by my students, I do not become infuriated when some students refer to me as a no-good. Many students do make absurd and unrelenting demands on teachers, parents, and peers. In their demands, they specify, in almost absolute propositions, the dimensions and requirements of an interpersonal encounter. As stated by some students, these demands require parents, teachers, and school administrators to "be genuine," "be authentic," "be real"; in the words of some students, "If you are not real, you are a shit." Instead, a student would be better off to say, "It would be nice if you older people were genuine, honest, authentic, and, ultimately, perfect, but since you are fallible, the best I can do is try to induce you to change and accept you even if you decide to remain unchanged." Moreover, the student might say, "If it is your desire to be neurotic, authoritarian, bigoted, and prejudiced, you have every right to be that way. But, I cannot and will not be that way; nor will I demand that you love and approve of me totally. I will live in spite of you and perhaps I'll mature in different ways." If ultimately internalized, these responses would be much more appropriate, much more logical and much more emotionally satisfying than the previous demands expressed by the students.

> *Irrational Idea Two:* One is only worthwhile if he is completely competent and nearly perfect in all that he attempts—or at least in one major area.

Many of our youth are obsessed with the belief that they must be perfect or highly accomplished in several areas of life. They must be as beautiful or more beautiful, more "freaky," or more brilliant than the average person. Their choice of a boyfriend, girlfriend, or group must fit some nearly perfect ideal.

Compulsive attempts by persons to achieve such states of near-perfection generally are associated with excessive anxiety. Persons who rigidly hold beliefs of this order generally underestimate, devaluate, and dismiss many of their fine achievements and strive endlessly for more perfection; they eventually become neurotically calculating, deliberating, and manipulating. Moreover, they defend and justify their actions with arguments like the Protestant Ethic. Ironically, when these people acquire the benefits of their realized achievements, they are very rarely satisfied. Sooner or later, it occurs to them that while they were spending virtually all their energy scheming, conniving, and aspiring, they lost sight of many other potentially meaningful life experiences.

Several of my own clients have expressed their dire needs for perfection—and achievement—in simple sentences: "I need and must develop a meaningful (perfect) relationship with someone;" "I cannot settle for less than the highest standards of performance in myself or in others;" "I must get into graduate school because one can't make it in this world without a Ph.D.;" "Look, if I don't associate myself with significant campus activity groups, I will not be considered for a top job when I graduate from college." Although such sentences do not necessarily reflect neurotic disturbances, they do imply a sort of grandiosity. Moreover, they may be good indicators of neurotic tendencies—especially when the failure to achieve, or achievement itself, results in self-defeating emotions and actions.

Neurotic proclivities toward achievement or perfection need not always be directed toward business or academic ends but may be observed in the striving of men and women to be paragons of masculinity or feminity. Quite often, for the young as well as for the old, one's masculine or feminine identity hinges upon one's power to attract others sexually. The process of striving for sexual activity as well as the sexual act itself are powerful symbols of masculinity or femininity in contemporary Western society. Perhaps too often, one's sexual accomplishments, defined in terms of the frequency, the intensity, and the duration of the sex act, easily become one's index of worth or worthlessness.

For example, a twenty-year-old male client told me that it was necessary for him to have sexual relationships with most of the girls he dated or else he felt terribly inadequate and depressed. He indicated further that he would tell a girl just about anything she wanted to hear if such revelations would lead to sex. One of his most successful strategies was to convince each girl that he wanted a meaningful and fulfilling relationship in which sex was a necessary but not a sufficient condition. This client was confused about the reasons for his severe depression, for when I asked him why he became disturbed when he did not get what he wanted, he replied, "Because she wouldn't give it to me." I responded, "Just because she refused your body means that you automatically became upset?" "Yes, that's right; that is absolutely correct." I replied immediately, "That is absolutely bullshit." Upon a more penetrating analysis of the client's concern, we soon discovered that much of his self-image was dependent upon the number of sexual encounters he could experience within a given time frame. In short, this client soon learned that his sense of sexual or male inadequacy was due not to the girls' refusal of his body but to his stupid, self-defeating belief that he would only be masculine or "good" if he could sleep with virtually every girl he dated. The client soon admitted that after he did have sex he wasn't sure whether he enjoyed the act. After a few sessions, the client discerned for himself that his inauthentic actions towards the opposite sex inhibited sexually satisfying relationships. Simply by attacking vigorously this client's fascistic sexual beliefs, I was able to assist him in acquiring the philosophy that sex is a delightful experience and is even more delightful when one is not obsessed with the idea that he must drive every girl into ecstasy (the idea that he must be sexually perfect). Why? Very simple. When one is obsessed with the idea of being sexually perfect, this idea prevents him from fully appreciating and focusing upon the more exciting, arousing aspects inherent in a sexual relationship.

Irrational Idea Three: Certain people are evil, wicked, or villains, and they should be severely reprimanded, blamed, and punished for their evil ways.

In our present youth culture there seems to be a greater acceptance, a greater tolerance of a variety of behavioral and philosophical styles. The phrase "live and let live" is not considered dated among the young; it is heard today as "do your own thing." Traditional moral and ethical codes, while still present, are seriously questioned. In evidence are the beginnings of a new moral thrust, a more personal morality. Yet in spite of noticeable rational trends in society in general — and in our youth specifically — one still observes needless and excessive prejudice, hostility, aggression, and hate directed towards specific persons, groups, and institutions.

Negative attitudinal or emotional states of persons that are expressed outwardly in the form of excessive blame and punishment of others are inspired by one's personal expectations or society's expectations. The idea has been perpetuated that certain persons or groups are the cause of the moral decay and the upheaval in our present-day society and that these same people or groups must be punished or eradicated.

Interestingly enough, people tend to blame others as the source of their own psychological disturbances. A neurotic mother may blame her drug addict son or daughter for her personal condition. The young addict then counters her thoughts by blaming his mother for his or her addiction. Wives and husbands blame and punish each other for their unsuccessful marriages. Students blame professors for their poor grades. However, excessive and indiscriminate blame and punishment are manifestations of emotional disturbance.

It is silly and self-defeating for one to express his anger and hostility in the form of undue blame and punishment because he risks the same kind of treatment from others, and, more importantly, if he tends to blame himself needlessly for his own imperfections, he may subsequently experience guilt, anxiety, or depression. A person would be much better off if he would accept fully the fact that human beings are prone to error biologically, psychologically, and sociologically. Because one is imperfect or fails at some task does not mean that he is absolutely worthless or that he will never succeed in life.

While counseling a nineteen-year-old, self-admitted, homosexual male, I noticed that the client vigorously, grandiosely, and with much hostility blamed society in general for his homosexual behavior and, more specifically, blamed his over-indulging mother and passive-aggressive father: "It is their fault that I am the way I am and there is no way that I or anyone else can do anything about my homosexuality. They made me this way. The very thought of my parents and the way they treated me still makes me depressed."

The client would not for one moment consider the possibility that much of the emotional disturbance which led to his homosexual practices was rooted in his own prejudiced, biased, and self-blaming thoughts. After several intensive counseling sessions, I was able to convince the client that blaming others for his own disturbance was not in his best interest, even though those others may have had a significant influence on his thinking, feeling, and behaving. The client was shown that while his parents may be neurotic themselves, he would be better off accepting rather than punishing or blaming them for their ignorance. Moreover, there would be little chance of changing the parents' lifestyle. Whether they would or would not change basically was irrelevant anyhow because they alone were not the most immediate cause of their son's behavior. By blaming others, the client, perhaps unconsciously, had avoided confronting the more relevant and significant factors causing and maintaining his homosexuality. Blaming others was one convenient strategy, among others, the client had devised to deny his underlying feelings of rejection by members of both sexes.

The client believed that to be rejected by others was a catastrophe; nothing could be worse. Since he had experienced a conditional type of acceptance by other homosexuals, who supposedly understood his feelings, he had concluded that the gay world was for him even though he was disturbed by his homosexuality as well as by some of the neurotic demands placed upon him by his gay friends. The client was shown that his illogical fears about being rejected were based upon faulty evidence. I did not accept as the most convincing evidence for the client's avoidance of intimate contact with females the rejection he had experienced by them two or three times in the past; I would not have accepted this argument even if he had been rejected one hundred times.

Why is it senseless to blame others and punish them too severely for their wrong doings? For one thing, excessive and indiscriminate blame and punishment are not the most effective means of problem-solving. A good testimonial to this fact is our inefficient penal institutions which serve only to reinforce and perpetuate criminal competence. Those who do punish and blame others excessively often overlook in others many of the positive qualities which ought to be reinforced but rarely are. In the final analysis, when people perform "wrong" or "immoral" acts, it is because of some emotional disturbance or stupidity. Consequently, it may be more logical to try to induce such people to act more reasonably or in ways that would be more self-enhancing than self-defeating. It is far more helpful to try to change aggravating or stupid behavior by stimulating and reinforcing more appropriate behavioral alternatives instead of repeatedly and antagonistically blaming or punishing.

Irrational Idea Four: It is terrible, horrible, and catastrophic when life's situations are not exactly the way one would like them to be.

The belief that it is terrible or catastrophic when one does not get what he wants out of life seems to be held by an overwhelming majority of children, youth, and adults. A tenacious belief of this sort is a typical cause of personal unhappiness and misery. Persons who overcatastrophize their frustrations and disappointments often become outwardly hostile and aggressive or inwardly depressed.

Counselors and therapists listen to their clients time and again express this belief in many ways. For instance, the college student might say, "The reason I am disturbed and nervous is that I wanted an "A" in your course and you didn't give it to me." The high-school student may say, "You son of a bitch, I'm going to beat the shit out of you for stealing my girlfriend away." The frustrated wife says to her husband, "I am depressed because I have to take care of you (the husband) and the kids and have no time for myself." In return, the frustrated husband angrily says, "Our marriage is doomed or is a failure because you (the wife) don't have sex with me upon demand." The not-so-handsome teenage boy thinks, "I am no good, and it's horrible that I can't have the pretty girls to ball like all the other guys." And we hear the twenty-year-old fat girl demand, "I should be skinny; it is terrible and awful that I am fat. Because I am fat, I am bad and depressed."

Even though most people normally are disappointed when they don't get what they want out of life, this fourth idea is irrational for several reasons:

1. While it may be naturally annoying to a person when he does not get something he really wants, it is only catastrophic when the person believes or thinks this is so. A more rational way of thinking about frustrating events follows.

   a. "I don't like being called dirty names like 'mother-fucker' or 'bastard.' So the next time I am called by one of these names, I will confront calmly the name caller with my thoughts on the matter and try to induce him to stop. If I can't change him, it might be unfortunate, but it is certainly not catastrophic. Sticks and stones may break my bones, but there is no way dirty names or psychological insults can really get me down unless I allow them to do so."

   A more irrational thought goes something like this:

   b. "I don't like being called a 'mother-fucker' or a 'bastard' by that person. He doesn't have the right to act that way toward me. He is making me out as a no-good and I couldn't stand being thought of as a no-good even though in many respects, deep down, I believe I am. If this situation does not change, I can't possibly be happy."

The first sentence in this self-talk sequence may be associated with some regret or unhappiness, but if the self-talk stops, the person will not become inordinately upset emotionally. It is only when he moves to the next set of sentences, in which he adopts a self-pitying and catastrophic philosophy, that emotional reactions, such as depression, anger, or hostility, are likely to result.

2. If a person persistently turns his frustrations into a catastrophe, he is less likely to focus on appropriate problem-solving strategies to surmount them. Why? Simply because he is spending most of his time lamenting, feeling sorry for himself, and identifying with other miserably unhappy persons and thereby undesirably reinforcing himself. Even though other persons may act stupidly, unfairly, and insanely toward a person, the best that person can do is to try to change that situation, even though he may be temporarily upset. If one cannot change the unfairness or stupidity of others, he need not demand dogmatically or persistently that those persons change and remain emotionally upset because he does not get his way.

3. Whether reality is or is not what one would like it to be, it is more desirable to accept it when it cannot be changed. Even though one has been frustrated in his attempts to achieve certain goals in life, frustration will rarely kill or defeat him unless he allows it to do so (Ellis and Harper, 1961).

Irrational Idea Five: External events are the cause of most human behavior and people have little or no ability to control their own happiness or their own sorrows and disturbances.

Today, there is an unsusally strong tendency for unhappy persons to ascribe the cause of their unhappiness to other persons, institutions, or events. It is a common belief that individuals have no control over their thoughts, feelings, and actions associated with undesirable political, economic, social, or personal events.

For instance, many of our college students are concerned about American involvement in Southeast Asia. A number of students have complained to me that they have become extremely upset with the political, economic, and social direction of the United States. The responses of these students have ranged from a lethargic lack of action to violent disruptions on college campuses. In many instances, students have constructively acted by committing themselves to enhancing the well-being of the society at large, but others have responded in emotionally self-defeating ways. For instance, one client indicated to me that she became depressed and was driven to the use of drugs because society is basically hostile, citing as an example the war and racism. Specifically, I asked her just how society magically caused her emotional disturbance and excessive drug usage. She said, "Because the majority of the society are racist-imperialistic pigs who are trying to do the rest of us in." I responded, "It seems to me that you may be upsetting yourself by defining certain events as personally catastrophic, terrible, awful, and so forth. And you may be telling yourself, 'When things don't go the way I would like them to go, I can't stand it.' " I replied, "You then feel depressed. Now, that's a hell of a lot different from laying it on the society exclusively. What you say the society is laying on you is really what you are laying on yourself. I would agree that these are annoying aspects of this society and that you might wish to change these things, but can you really be a creatively effective change agent if you are constantly depressed or high on drugs?"

In general, events external to the individual, although often inconveniencing, rarely are the direct cause of unhappiness. Exceptions to this may be found in environments where there is evidence of extreme poverty, hunger, and economic deprivation. Many minority persons — Blacks, Chicanos, Puerto Ricans — normally and naturally respond to deficit conditions with frustration, aggression, or depression. But for the majority of society, there are few deficit physiological, safety, and economic needs to overwhelm the individual. Of course, if a person suffers injury or pain as a result of a physical attack or accident, one can argue effectively that this event is indeed a direct cause of the person's condition. Psychological attacks, unlike physical attacks, are only emotionally upsetting and that is only when the person who receives the attack defines it as awful or catastrophic. If one is to minimize needless emotional arousal associated with psychological attacks, it may be advisable to accept the attacker in spite of what he says or does; understand that most persons who indiscriminately attack him may be emotionally disturbed or stupid themselves; understand and accept that their attacks have nothing to do with his own personal worth; accept that other persons have the right to say what they want to say; and if it is at all desirable to change these persons, devise and implement reasonable strategies to do so calmly.

As an example of dealing with psychological attacks, one can simply ignore them.

Irrational Idea Six: A person should be overly preoccupied with fear and anxiety about events that are uncertain or potentially dangerous.

Fear and anxiety are closely related phenomena but differ in at least one major respect. Although both are experienced as apprehensive excitations which signal some impending real or imagined danger, anxiety is a special case of exaggerated fear. Rarely the result of an objective appraisal of external stimuli, anxiety is a response to highly biased and distorted interpretive-evaluative thinking. In short, a person becomes unnecessarily anxious when he projects that some event will occur which will bring psychological misfortune.

People in western society quite often become anxious over what they think other people think about them. Therefore, if the notion of anxiety is examined closely, one observes that anxiety has an interpersonal dimension. An instance of the interpersonal aspect in anxiety reactions is obvious in persons who become physically or emotionally upset prior to taking examinations. For example, one Ph.D. student asked for an appointment with me about two weeks before his general examinations so that he could discuss the rationale and purposes of Ph.D. examinations. In that hour, he gave a scholarly analysis and critique of the entire system of Ph.D. examinations. In many respects — although not all — I agreed with him but noticed while he was talking, his breathing became more rapid and he was perspiring. I asked him if there was anything else bothering him. He disclosed that he was horrified about taking his examinations and complained about many sleepless nights, great irritability, and inability to think about important things. As there was little doubt in my mind that the student was well prepared for the examinations, a lack of adequate preparation should not have been a cause for his anxiety. Instead, later in the session the student admitted that his fears were reactions to his thoughts that his father would not accept him if he failed his examinations. Quite compulsively, the student imagined scenes of his father's scorn and rejection if he did not excel academically.

Most of us are fearful and sometimes anxious about such things as the possibility of failing or not performing well on a given task. And such fear is quite normal, when it is a response to a situation that is laden with real dangers to the physical well-being of a person (i.e., a severe hurricane warning). But even in such normal and objective situations, a person does not have to exaggerate his fear or dwell incessantly upon it. He would be better off to acknowledge the fear, to accept it as an uncomfortable emotional state, and to take the necessary constructive actions to counteract the real or potential danger. Anxiety that is intense and perpetual often leads one to inappropriate behaviors which interfere with the person's ability to function adequately in social situations.

In situations where a person predicts accurately that something unfortunate will occur but cannot prevent it (a divorce, financial hardship, etc.), he does not have to focus on the event and catastrophize endlessly about it. He may experience perfectly normal sadness or unhappiness temporarily, which need not interfere with other growth-enhancing behavior (relating well with others, working effectively at his job, etc.).

Irrational Idea Seven: Life difficulties and responsibilities are easier to avoid than they are to face.

In *Escape From Freedom* (1941), Eric Fromm depicts the ease with which a man avoids freedom by escaping into conformity and dependence upon others rather than facing the difficult task of affirming his own sense of identity and thinking for himself. Many believe that it is easier in the short run to escape problematic situations, such as a broken engagement, a divorce, a death, or a physical or mental condition, by engaging in the excessive use of drugs, alcohol, sex, or fantasy. But such predilections towards avoidance and escape only reinforce the idea that one is capable of acting constructively and that if one does try, he will probably fail, thereby proving that he need not confront the personal conflicts at all.

When the translation of one's thoughts and feelings into constructive actions rarely occurs, it becomes increasingly difficult for one to develop a close identification with an unavoidable part of the human condition which is pain and discomfort. Moreover, learning is stifled if one fails to submit his ideas or philosophies about life to the empirical test.

A young female college student of about nineteen years related to me that she was deeply depressed over her fear of telling a steady boyfriend that she no longer loved him and wanted to break up. I asked how long she had had these feelings and if she had attempted at all to tell her boyfriend about them. She indicated that she had felt this way for about six months but hadn't been able to say anything because she didn't want to hurt him. She thought it was better if she suffered. In simple ABC talk, the girl was saying something like this:

(A) There is a boy I have dated for about one year and he was the only boy I dated until I met another guy.

(B) I would like to leave my boyfriend for this other guy but I can't bring myself to do it because I don't want to hurt him. I would rather suffer than see him suffer. I don't like where I am and want to get out but I just don't know how. Why do I feel this way? Why can't he leave me? He doesn't deserve this. I am really awful—bad; I can't tell him. I can't stand to hurt anyone.

(C) I feel really depressed and rotten.

I asked her why she had a difficult time expressing her thoughts and feelings to the boyfriend. Essentially, she said, "Because I just can't. We made an emotional commitment to one another; there was sexual intimacy and what I thought to be a total commitment. I haven't lived up to my commitment."

This example, I think is a dilemma experienced by many persons involved in close heterosexual relationships but do not choose to act reasonably, constructively, and authentically. After five intensive counseing sessions, this girl decided that maybe she had made a mistake by encouraging a relationship which she did not really want in the first place and in trying to convince herself of the authenticity and uniqueness of that relationship. Moreover, she was able to see that just because she had made a mistake, she did not have to blame herself needlessly or condemn herself to a life of martyrdom. Also, she realized that it would be in her best interest to have a calm discussion with her boyfriend during which she would share her thoughts. I assured her that she could expect the young man to react somewhat emotionally but that in the long run, he would be better off if she was honest about her feelings.

Two weeks after the fifth counseling session, the girl came to see me and told me she had confronted the boyfriend calmly and honestly with her decision to date several boys rather than just one. Although the boy was somewhat upset, he agreed that such a decision was in their mutual best interest. She also indicated that she felt very clean about having faced a rather difficult situation.

Frequently, high school and college students exhibit minimal self-discipline related to academic performance. Students complain often to their counselors and teachers that they cannot concentrate efficiently on their assignments and would rather socialize. Even though study is often an arduous and boring task, most students do persist long enough to pass their examinations or to master the subject matter of a given course. Still, we encounter many students who fail to discipline themselves in organizing and allotting time to prepare adequately for their courses. The consequence of such inertia is often low grades or failure. And, interestingly enough, failure in school, rather than reflecting low intelligence or some organic brain deficiency, is in large measure a matter of deficiency in self-control over the study situation.

Students often will admit they have not learned the art and science of concentrating or focusing their attention on academic matters. The question, of course, is simple, "How do these seemingly unmotivated, lethargic students become motivated to develop the necessary skills for self-control and learning?" Systematic techniques have been developed and employed successfully to induce students to perform more effectively in academic settings (Premack, 1965; Robinson, 1946; Tosi, Briggs, Morily, 1971). Some of these methods are discussed in chapters that follow. But the main key is hard and persistent effort and work—period. One must accept the fact that he must spend time—sometimes painful time—working both at his studies and to overcome his lack of control. Literally, he must force himself to work.

Recently, I have been trying to understand some new statistical concepts which are relatively foreign to me. During a doctoral student's dissertation examination, I had some questions about her statistical analysis. Although she responded quite brilliantly to my inquiry, there was one problem; I didn't understand her answer. Following the examination, I asked a renowned psychometrician at Ohio State University, who was also a member of the doctoral student's committee, just how long it takes one to understand the particular statistic if he hasn't had the previous training. I was surprised when he said, in essence, "When I received my Ph.D. in 1929, most of the statistical concepts used in psychological research were not invented. As a matter of fact, today I teach just about two percent of what I learned during graduate school. Ninety-eight percent of what I presently know came after my degree and was acquired through hours and hours of study — as a matter of fact — years. You know, if I read an article in *Psychometrika* (a psychological statistical journal) I rarely understand it on the first try. I spend thirty or forty hours working through some of the mathematical equations given in that article and end up running the new analysis five or six times on various sets of data." He further added, "I had to learn virtually all of the mathematical derivations of statistics after my Ph.D. I worked, worked, and worked."

During our conversation, I thought to myself, "So I *should* understand thoroughly this statistical concept after reading one article—what grandiosity. Now if I really want to learn these concepts, I had better adopt the philosophy that I had better work a lot harder."

Ellis and Harper (1961) suggest that evading life's difficulties and self-responsibilities tends to result, in the long run, in less rewarding activities and decreased self-acceptance. Human beings are fallible, and one aspect of their fallibility is a normal biological tendency to resist constructive or reasonable action. If a person is to acquire self-discipline, he must accept many personally distasteful factors and act constructively in spite of them. Literally, he may have to force himself into action and hard work. Of course, excessive self-discipline can be as self-defeating as lack of self-discipline. In addition, Ellis and Harper warn against becoming too self-disciplining and self-punishing for the sake of receiving some magical reward.

Irrational Idea Eight: A person's past is all-important to one's present behavior, and because certain events once strongly influenced one's life, these events will indefinitely do so.

Determining psychologies, such as orthodox psychoanalytic and behavioristic theories, have given the impression that man's present behavior is largely a function of early childhood experiences (traumas, unresolved unconscious conflicts) or early conditioning. Certainly, in the formation of one's existing cognitions, affections, and behaviors, his past learnings, as well as certain hereditary predispositions, play a vital part. But just because man is influenced significantly by his past conditioning, he need not continue to be forever influenced in the same manner. The negative effects of some past experiences, it must be understood, are not perpetuated magically by themselves over time but are symbolized, sustained, and perpetuated by the person himself in the form of prejudiced self-verbalizations. This being the case, it is possible for a person to alter such pernicious internalized cognitive/affective states by learning to challenge and to contradict them and by replacing them with more reasonable thoughts, feelings, and actions. Thus, a person can decondition himself and minimize to his satisfaction most of his perniciously displeasing influences of his past.

A male client (twenty-seven years of age) expressed intense anxiety over taking a new job, following the completion of his Master's degree in Business Administration. He believed that he would fall drastically short of meeting the job's expectations because of some bad experiences he had had on some previous jobs. Briefly, his idea was: "Because I performed poorly on my first real job several years ago, I will always continue to perform that way on any new job. I am destined to fail." When I asked him just what the evidence was for his conclusion he said, "Well the past—isn't that the best predictor of the future?" To his idea, I said, "Yes, perhaps, assuming you haven't done anything to modify your past thinking and believing. You can easily perpetuate the past and even prove some of your existing stupid ideas by continually thinking and acting stupidly. But since you are now in counseling, you can begin, or have already begun, to conquer some of your emotionally stupid ideas."

In only a matter of a few counseling sessions, the client did attack rather successfully his fear of failing and his avoidance tendencies. With the counselor's active assistance, he took the new job rather than avoiding it and made great progress in applying the ABC method of thinking to his fears. Presently on the job, the client exudes much more self-confidence in his ability to perform. Most importantly, however, he is acquiring the philosophy that it would not be horrible or catastrophic if he should fail once again, although he would be happier if his job performance was commensurate with his ability and skill.

> *Irrational Idea Nine:*   People and things in this society should be different from the way they are and it is horrible or catastrophic that correct solutions to the problems that plague society are not immediate.

Domestic and international social, political, and economic crises have characterized the 1960s and early 1970s. There were racial riots in major cities, violence on the college campuses, political assassinations, emerging awareness of extreme poverty and deprivation among Puerto Ricans, Blacks, Appalachian whites, and other minority groups, the rise of the drug culture, increased divorce rates, which indicate a break-up of the traditional family, and an economic recession.

One cannot easily escape or deny that he has strong feelings about the world he lives in today. People, especially our youth, are legitimately concerned. Youth today have assumed a more meaningful and active role in reforming and reconstructing our society than ever before. Emerging is a "new assertiveness" which symbolizes an openness and direct confrontation with issues basic to man's existence. Openness, confrontation, and constructive action, the indications of this "new assertiveness," are potentially the powerful undergirdings for more creative and humanistic solutions to our contemporary social problems.

It is to be hoped that we are moving into an era in which persons will deemphasize symbols and be more responsive to the personal meanings or interpretations they ascribe to symbols. Only then can we hope to understand the meaning of the human condition.

In spite of some justification for optimism, these recent trends of youth towards openness may not always be rational or authenic. Many of our youth, like their adult counterparts, still become needlessly disturbed when things are not exactly the way they want them to be and because perfect solutions are not immediate. For instance, some who demonstrate for the legalization of drugs become highly disturbed because the system will not accept immediately their philosophy. Many gay liberationists believe it is catastrophic that "straight society" will not accept homosexuality as a legitimate life style.

The undercurrent of many of the demands of youth on society may represent a "short-term hedonistic philosophy." The philosophy is something like this, "I want what I want upon demand and if I don't get it, it is horrible and terrible and I can't stand it." A more productive philosophy, one which balances a short-term hedonic philosophy with a long-term hedonic philosophy, would sound like this, "I would like to see a liberalization of the drug laws, for this is my value and conviction and I will work to bring this about, realizing that some time may be necessary to accomplish this task. If my hopes were fulfilled tomorrow, it would be nice; if not 'tough shit!' "

One should keep the following items in mind when he wishes to contradict Irrational Idea Nine (Ellis and Harper, 1961):

1. People and things are, the way they are and while it might be nice theoretically if they were different and to our liking, this is no reason for them to be different upon demand.
2. Becoming needlessly upset and concerned about people and events can easily keep one from focusing upon his own growth and development. It is easy to avoid one's own concerns by becoming preoccupied with the lives of others.
3. Since there are rarely perfect and right solutions to human problems, one would be better off thinking in terms of the advantages and disadvantages of alternative solutions.[1]

Irrational Idea Ten: Maximum human happiness can best be achieved by inaction, inertia, passivity, and uncommittedly enjoying oneself.

Effective living encompasses doing, acting, feeling, loving, creating, and thinking (Ellis and Harper, 1961). Passivity, inaction, and laziness, while not inherently pernicious forms of existence, are growth inhibiting. While man's cognitive functioning, or his ability to think and to think about his thinking, is a virtue and a necessary function, it is also often misused. That is, a person can easily consider the question of his existence in the world solely as an academic or intellectual matter about himself without committing himself to constructive actions. Or he may test out his ideas of hypothesis about himself or the world intellectually but never in real life. Ideally, or perhaps reasonably and realistically, effective living, existing, and becoming involve the reasonable and the constructive affirmation of one's thoughts, ideas, and feelings. Unreasonable or compulsive focusing on cognitive activity at the exclusion of affective and behavioral activity can leave a person lopsided or "in his head." Rational thinking and believing about oneself is of significant importance to man's growth if it serves as a springboard to positive feelings and emotions and ultimately to his self-actualization.

Although many persons appear to be cognitively lopsided, still others appear affectively lopsided. Today's encounter-group movement is an alleged attempt to balance cognitive and affective activity. Encounter groups can be indeed useful and effective in helping persons attend to and become more aware of their emotions and feelings and to express these affective states physically or verbally. Unfortunately, encounter-group experiences also may facilitate compulsive focusing on affect which can be just as defeating as compulsive cognizing. A priority on affect may be associated with a person's failure to act reasonably and may simply reinforce "emotional gut-level responses" as a sole guide to action. Thus, a person may passively and uncommitedly enjoy himself through heightened affect (joy, euphoria, sensuality) while, at the same time, deluding himself into thinking that he is growing when he is not.

There are also those who espouse a dogmatic "behavioristic position" emphasizing effective actions and deemphasizing rational thinking and emotions. This position can lead to compulsive strivings for a person to be an effective role player or actor in social situations so he may maximize personal rewards from others. However, in this approach, there is the debilitating possibility that a peron may look nice or act in accordance with prescribed roles but be emotionally disturbed. For example, the organization man seems to suggest a "behaviorally lopsided person."

Ellis and Harper (1961) suggest that Irrational Idea Ten is self-defeating for the following reasons:

1. Man is a species of animal who is not particularly happy when he is inert. Passive or vicarious experiences, such as reading, watching TV, or attending lectures, while quite entertaining, and enjoyable, may lead to feelings of alienation if they are an exclusive diet.

2. Most persons are highly gratified when they are involved in complex, absorbing, and challenging work or play.
3. Long-term inaction or inertia may be associated with depression. Activity, on the other hand, is a means of alleviating depression. But high levels of activity or manic behavior sustained for long periods of time can be equally self-defeating. Calm, undramatic and persistent absorption in achieving some long-range creative goal is generally a very satisfying kind of activity as opposed to compulsive manic strivings.
4. Constructive action often is required to break the vicious cycle of self-defeating behavior or habits. The greater one's inertia and lethargic tendencies, the greater the probability that one will remain in those states. A lethargic philosophy, when it is based on fear of failure, is an impediment to self-regard.

Farquhar and Lowe (1968) have added twelve more irrational ideas to Ellis's list. They also present the rational alternatives to the irrational ideas.

1. The idea that each individual has a discoverable, internally consistent "self" and that one should strive to always behave in accord with "self"—instead of the idea that each individual is a complex-composite of all emotions and that the true spice of living is accepting and experiencing one's emotional and intellectual shifts.
2. The idea that one's worth as a person is directly related to one's objectively discernible productivity—instead of the idea that one's worth to himself rests in his aliveness and in his capacity to enjoy living.
3. The idea that there is a hierarchy of values and that secondary processes, i.e., the enjoyment of music, art, and literature, are inherently superior to primary processes, i.e., physical passion, eating, etc.—instead of the idea that all nondestructive drives and emotions are a source of both immediate and long-term pleasure and goodness in living.
4. The idea that anger is automatically bad, obscene, and destructive and that one should always curb his anger—instead of the idea that anger is a normal human emotion which can be cleansing and nurturing and that one should work at expressing anger as a communication of current feelings without attacking the personal worth and security of others.
5. The idea that people are very fragile and that one should always keep his thoughts to himself in order to avoid hurting others—instead of the idea that sharing one's perceptions can often be one of the most direct expressions of love a human can make.

6. The idea that it is better to give than to receive—rather than the idea that meaningful human relationships are based upon giving and receiving and that the exclusion of either is damaging to the relationship and the individual.

7. The idea that one should always try to please others and, if necessary, forego his own pleasures and desires in doing so—instead of the idea that one has the "right to live" and to enjoy himself and that consistent self-denial usually results in bitterness.

8. The idea that when one receives the disapproval of others, it invariably means that one is wrong and bad—instead of the idea that another's disapproval is simply an expression of his own emotional state and has relatively little meaning about anyone else.

9. The idea that there are certain absolute and universal definitions of such things as happiness, success, morality, love, etc.—instead of the ideas that man is free and that each individual experiences these phenomena according to his own self-definition.

10. The idea that happiness, pleasure, fulfillment, and growth can only occur in the presence of others and that being alone is the worst possible human condition—rather than the idea that happiness, pleasure, etc. can be experienced alone as well as with others and that being alone at times is a desirable human experience.

11. The idea that the emergence of any sign of hostility, anger, aggression, or fear is a sign of broad, deep-seated problems—rather than the idea that one should first consider that they may be temporary or realistic expressions of inner emotions or feelings.

12. The idea that there is always some perfect solution to human problems and that one should strive to find this solution—rather than the idea that many decisions and solutions are a compromise between what people want and what they do not want.[1]

a measure of irrational thinking

In 1968, B. J. Hartman constructed a self-administered, objectively-scored, diagnostic instrument reported to be used to measure specific levels of irrational thinking. The instrument was known as the *Personal Belief Inventory*. Initially, Dr. Hartman reviewed existing literature and pooled 135 preliminary items. These items were subsequently administered

[1]W. Farquhar and J. Lowe, "A List of Ellis's Irrational Ideas" (Unpublished paper, Michigan State University, 1968).

to 500 college students and analyzed. The result was the sixty-item PBI. With a maximum score of 300 and a minimum of sixty (60), the PBI is constructed so that the higher the individual's score, the more irrational his thoughts can be said to be. A slightly revised version of the *Personal Beliefs Inventory* follows.

chart 1
personal beliefs inventory[2]

The following items represent certain beliefs and opinions people have in general. If you agree or disagree with an item indicate the extent of that agreement or disagreement by assigning the following values to each responses: *disagree very much,* one point; *disagree slightly,* two points; *agree slightly,* three points; *agree very much,* four points; *totally agree,* five points. There are no correct or incorrect answers. Please respond to each item.

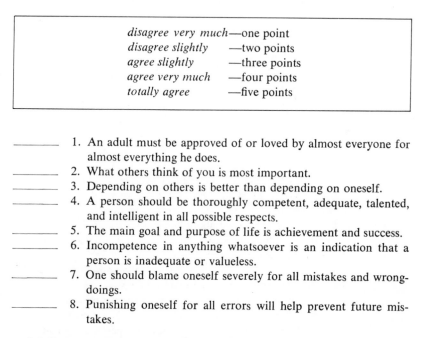

> *disagree very much*—one point
> *disagree slightly*   —two points
> *agree slightly*   —three points
> *agree very much*   —four points
> *totally agree*   —five points

_____ 1. An adult must be approved of or loved by almost everyone for almost everything he does.

_____ 2. What others think of you is most important.

_____ 3. Depending on others is better than depending on oneself.

_____ 4. A person should be thoroughly competent, adequate, talented, and intelligent in all possible respects.

_____ 5. The main goal and purpose of life is achievement and success.

_____ 6. Incompetence in anything whatsoever is an indication that a person is inadequate or valueless.

_____ 7. One should blame oneself severely for all mistakes and wrong-doings.

_____ 8. Punishing oneself for all errors will help prevent future mistakes.

[2]B.J. Hartman, "Sixty Revealing Questions for Twenty Minutes," *Rational Living* 3 (1968): 7-8. Reprinted by permission of the journal.

chart 1 (continued)

> *disagree very much*—one point
> *disagree slightly*   —two points
> *agree slightly*   —three points
> *agree very much*   —four points
> *totally agree*   —five points

_____ 9. A person should blame others for their mistaken or bad behavior.

_____ 10. One should spend considerable time and energy trying to reform others.

_____ 11. One can best help others by criticizing them and sharply pointing out the error of their ways.

_____ 12. It is natural to get upset by the errors and stupidities of others.

_____ 13. Because a certain thing once strongly affected one's life, it should indefinitely affect it.

_____ 14. Because a person was once weak and helpless, he must always remain so.

_____ 15. Because parents or society taught acceptance of certain traditions, one must go on accepting these traditions.

_____ 16. If things are not the way one would like them to be, it is a catastrophe.

_____ 17. Other people should make things easier for us and help with life's difficulties.

_____ 18. No one should have to put off present pleasures for future gains.

_____ 19. Avoiding life's difficulties and self-responsibilities is easier than facing them.

_____ 20. Inertia and inaction are necessary and/or pleasant.

_____ 21. One should rebel against doing things, however necessary, if doing them is unpleasant.

_____ 22. Much unhappiness is externally caused or created by outside persons and events.

_____ 23. A person has virtually no control over his emotions and cannot help feeling bad on many occasions.

_____ 24. If something is or may be dangerous or injurious, one should be seriously concerned about it.

_____ 25. Worrying about a possible danger will help ward it off or decrease its effect.

_____ 26. Certain people are bad, wicked, or villainous and should be severely blamed and punished for their sins.

_____ 27. Maximum human happiness can be achieved by passively and uncommittedly "enjoying oneself."

_____ 28. Any job should be done thoroughly and perfectly if you do it at all.

chart 1 (continued)

> *disagree very much*—one point
> *disagree slightly* —two points
> *agree slightly* —three points
> *agree very much* —four points
> *totally agree* —five points

_____ 29. People should observe moral laws more strictly than they do.

_____ 30. I get annoyed at being held up by small rules and regulations.

_____ 31. I get impatient, and begin to fume and fret, when people delay me unnecessarily.

_____ 32. When I'm in a group, I'm always afraid I may say or do something foolish.

_____ 33. If you once start doing favors for people, they may just walk all over you.

_____ 34. I tend to do or say things I later hate myself for.

_____ 35. When things go badly, I tend to blame myself too much.

_____ 36. I feel that many people could be described as victims of circumstances beyond their control.

_____ 37. The trouble with many people is that they don't take things seriously enough.

_____ 38. For most questions there is one right answer, once a person has the facts.

_____ 39. People today have forgotten how to feel properly ashamed of themselves.

_____ 40. I set a high standard for myself and feel others should do the same.

_____ 41. Criticism makes me very nervous and anxious.

_____ 42. I often do whatever makes me feel good at the moment, even at the cost of some distant goal.

_____ 43. I am so touchy on some subjects that I can't talk about them.

_____ 44. A large number of people are guilty of bad sexual conduct.

_____ 45. Some of my family and/or friends have habits that bother and annoy me very much.

_____ 46. My feelings are easily hurt.

_____ 47. I feel self-conscious and uncomfortable when in the presence of those whom I consider to be my superiors.

_____ 46. I worry quite a bit over possible misfortune.

_____ 49. At times I think I am no good at all.

_____ 50. I often get excited or upset when things go wrong.

_____ 51. I shrink from facing a crisis or difficulty.

_____ 52. I have reason for feeling jealous of one or more members of my family.

_____ 53. It makes me angry and upset when other people interfere with my daily activity.

chart 1 (continued)

> disagree very much—one point
> disagree slightly —two points
> agree slightly —three points
> agree very much —four points
> totally agree —five points

———— 54. I often become depressed because of my own deficiencies or shortcomings.

———— 55. I often feel guilty because of the sins I have committed.

———— 56. I tend to become terribly upset and miserable when things are not the way I would like them to be.

———— 57. There is invariably a right, precise and perfect solution to human problems and it is catastrophic when this perfect solution isn't found.

———— 58. You owe obedience to your parents just because they are your parents.

———— 59. I tend to take myself and others too seriously.

———— 60. It is realistic to expect that there should be no incompatibility in marriage.

summary

In summary, Ellis's ten irrational ideas that cause and sustain emotional disturbances were discussed. Specific rational alternatives to these irrational beliefs were also introduced. Farquhar and Lowe's additions to Ellis's original ten irrational ideas were also included here as well as Hartman's *Personal Beliefs Inventory*, a measure of irrational thinking.

The next chapter, Rational-Emotive Techniques, discusses the methods RE counselors employ to intervene in the lives of their clients. It will be recalled from Chapter One that the aim of counseling is to facilitate the personal growth or self-realization of the client. To accomplish this, the RE interventions are designed specifically to assist the person in changing or modifying significantly those irrational ideas and beliefs, emotions, and behavior that obstruct or retard his growth.

four ✶ techniques in rational-emotive counseling

Although counseling and psychotherapeutic systems share many intervention strategies in common, every system of counseling and psychotherapy has an identifiable set of techniques and methods which differentiate it from other systems. Rational-emotive counseling theory is no exception. Many of the techniques exclusive to rational-emotive counseling are explicated in this chapter.

In accordance with the self-in-situation or person-in-environment model depicted in Chapter One, rational-emotive treatment strategies—singly and in combination with other, primarily behavioristic techniques—are intended to intervene in the cognitive, affective, and behavioral domains of the person. The techniques described in this chapter may easily be extended into the specific environmental conditions in which the person interacts.

Specifically, Ellis's ABC technique of analyzing and confronting emotional disturbances will be explored in this chapter. In combination with behavioristically oriented interventions, such as social modeling, assertive training, rational-emotive imagery, and systematic desensitization, the use of the ABC technique will be presented here. Moreover, the application of rational-emotive counseling or intervention strategies to outside of counseling situations will also be emphasized. Examples of RE interventions on problems and conflicts expressed by youth, such as self-assertiveness, academic achievement, personal worth, and emotional control, will be given.

the abc's of emotional control

It is not uncommon for people who experience unpleasant emotional states to blame others or things external to themselves as the cause for their intense feelings. Psychotherapists and counselors have heard from their clients countless laments such as: "I become depressed only when my husband is around; therefore, he is the cause of my depression." "My teacher makes me so mad that I can't study." "If it weren't for my girl-friend leaving me for another guy, I would not be as unhappy as I am now." "This classmate of mine called me a 'bastard' and I just boiled inside and then knocked him on his ass." "Because Jane loves me so much, she makes me happy." "Mary would not make it with me at the drive-in movie, and she hurt my feelings."

The idea that external events are the direct cause of one's emotional reactions and behavior is rooted in "magical thinking," such as in "devil worship," or in some strict deterministic psychophilosophical systems (logical positivism and behavioristic psychology). The notion that one's thinking, emoting, and behaving also is controlled exclusively by some divine power beyond man's control is typical of many fundamental religions.

For the most part, rational-emotive theory rejects those ideas that place man or the organism in the hands of mysterious forces. On the matter of emotional control, rational-emotive counselors hold the view that when a person experiences anger, depression, or happiness, he can be assured that he alone, or that he primarily, is in control of that experience (Maultsby, 1969).

By and large, Western society, despite its claims otherwise, has posed severe constraints to rational thought. For the most part, persons, while giving the appearance of being rational through verbal communication, give themselves away through emotional disturbances and self-defeating behavior. If individuals are to learn more reasonable ways of thinking, feeling, and behaving, it is desirable that they be taught or helped by someone who is relatively rational himself. Usually, such a helper is a psychotherapist, a counselor, a teacher, a minister, or some reasonable layman.

The following excerpt is an example of a counselor's introduction of a seventeen-year adolescent boy to the ABC theory of problem analysis and emotional disturbance. The client is typical in that he has not given such a notion much thought and tends to have difficulty understanding it in relation to a problem he is having—in this case, the problem of expressing his feelings towards a secret love. To clarify for the client a rational thought process, the counselor uses as content some of the more immediate dynamics of their relationship.

Counselor:	How long have you been secretly in love with Tonie?
Client:	Since I was in junior high — about a year and a half.
Counselor:	Gee, that must seem like a long time to have such intense feelings.
Client:	Yeah! I know.
Counselor:	I imagine those feelings hurt sometimes.
Client:	Yeah, they really do.
Counselor:	It must be tough for you to express to Tonie the feelings you have for her.
Client:	(Pause) . . . I can't do that.
Counselor:	Why?
Client:	Because.
Counselor:	Because why?
Client:	I don't know.
Counselor:	Have you ever thought about what prevents you from doing that?
Client:	Well, I guess!
Counselor:	What have you thought?
Client:	I am not sure.
Counselor:	You mean you have a difficult time sharing some of your thoughts on the mater with me?
Client:	I don't know. I don't think so.
Counselor:	It sounds to me like you are hurt and not too sure where that hurt comes from.
Client:	Well, I love Tonie and that hurts me.
Counselor:	I understand that you feel hurt, but I am not too sure how that necessarily follows love. It may be that part of what you love about Tonie involves desiring her and wanting her. And I could see that desiring her and not having her might result in hurt for you.
Client:	I do love her!
Counselor:	Yes, I do think you feel that way but if we are to make some sense out of what love is, it is necessary to come to grips with your definition of it.
Client:	(Pause. Looks at the counselor confused).
Counselor:	You look confused — like "What in the hell is he talking about — man, doesn't he know what love is?" Is that right?
Client:	I don't know.
Counselor:	Listen now. You have been coming here for three sessions and you keep giving me the same nonsense — "I don't know; I don't know what I am thinking. All I know is that I am secretly in love and it hurts me and gets me down." Now, I think we have established firmly the fact that you feel hurt and the fact that you are in love with Tonie, but we haven't established the fact that being secretly in love with Tonie is the cause of your hurt, have we now?

Client: I guess so.

Counselor: What do you mean, "I guess so"? Yes, I know. You don't
               know. Maybe one of the reasons you have never approached
               Tonie is because you don't know how she will react to you:
               "Oh, maybe she won't like my program." Right? And, don't
               tell me you don't know.

Client: You don't understand me. (Client directs hostility to the
               counselor.)

Counselor: The hell I don't. I understand that you don't like to be
               pushed or maybe put down. But am I really putting you
               down? Hell, no! But maybe that's how you are interpreting
               my behavior. Maybe we ought to examine just what is going
               on between the two of us, OK?

Client: I guess so.

Counselor: Good! Let's see if this analysis makes some sense. First,
               let's label my confronting you or pushing you as *(A)*. Second,
               let's label your thoughts or what you think about what I
               am doing as *(B)*. Third, let's label your feelings *(C)*, which in
               this case was some anger toward me.

Client: OK.

Counselor: Do you understand the differences between *(A)*, *(B)*, and
               (C) ?

Client: Yes.

Counselor: Are you sure?

Client: Yeah!

Counselor: Then explain the difference.

Client: Uh . . . I can't.

Counselor: OK. Let me spell out the whole thing again. This time I
               will diagram it on this paper. Follow me closely. The *(A)*
               stands for my behavior towards you — pushing, question-
               ing, disagreeing, etc. OK? The *(B)* stands for your thoughts
               about me — the *(A)*. OK?

Client: Yes.

Counselor: Good; the *(C)* stands for your feelings. In this case, your anger
               is towards me. I think you have to admit you did get a little
               mad at me.

Client: OK.

Counselor: I would guess that your analysis of this situation would be
               something like this. The counselor's behavior — *(A)* — was
               the cause of my anger — *(C)*. Right?

Client: Yeah!

Counselor: That's nonsense! Of course, you and most other human be-
               ings have a normal tendency to believe the *(A)* is the direct
               cause of *(C)*. Or, that someone else's actions which are di-
               rected towards you are the cause of your feelings. But, if

we examine the situation a little more closely, we would soon discover that *(A)* (the event external to you) is not the cause of *(C)* (your negative emotion) but the most direct cause of *(C)* would be *(B)* (your thoughts about *(A)*.

Client: Um! (a confused "Um").

Counselor: I pick up a little confusion on your part but that's OK. One of the reasons you are here is to learn more about yourself. But that means coming to grips with your thoughts, feelings, and actions. It seems like one of your problems is being able to understand your own thoughts at point B and how your thinking may have something to do with the way you feel and act.

rational-emotive modeling (rem)

Persons learn or acquire new behaviors under a variety of conditions and experiences which may be direct, simulated, or vicarious in nature. Bandura (1969), for one, has emphasized strongly that a person acquires many behaviors by simply imitating or observing the behavior of others. Moreover, imitative learning or social modeling is involved in the strengthening or weakening behaviors which already exists in a person's behavior repertoire and, also, in the facilitation of behaviors which have not been punished previously.

Bandura and Whalen (1966) believe that learning by means of social modeling or imitation does not necessarily involve externally reinforced performance. That is, a person may observe a model but perform no overt action which is reinforced by others. The modeled response on the observer's part occurs at a covert and cognitive representational level. The performance of observationally acquired responses may be governed by reinforcing events that are applied by external sources which are experienced vicariously or self-administered.

Rational-emotive counseling emphasizes the importance of the person's gaining greater control over himself and his environment. The importance of such external reinforcement from the environment as monetary rewards and social approval are not to be denied as having a relationship to one's behavior. But, ultimately, the person should learn ways of applying reinforcement to himself (self-reinforcement). One of the major goals of counseling is to help the client learn to make finer discriminations between those thoughts, feelings, and overt actions which are self-enhancing and those which are self-defeating. Another goal which logically follows is to assist the client to evaluate those discriminations in such a way that when he does act upon his rational thoughts and feelings, he evaluates his actions in positive terms. If he does make a mistake in judgment or action, he does not have to punish himself or negatively reinforce himself so severely that he systematically avoids appropriate actions and responsibilities. In other words, rational-emotive counseling teaches the client to accept his mistakes and to evaluate his inappropriate thoughts, feelings, and actions as not being in his best interest, although they are humanly and unavoidably natural. The client also is shown that negatively describing himself with such labels as "a louse," "a shit," "a no-good," or "an absolutely worthless idiot" will only lead to more self-defeating behavior. On the other hand, the client is taught to contradict such negative, self-defeating labels and thoughts and to emphasize instead positive self-reinforcing sentences and thoughts.

By now, one should recognize that rational-emotive counseling has a strong didactic component. The counselor should employ any device or audio-visual-experiential aid that will facilitate the client's learning effective and efficient ways of operating in his environment. Thus, social modeling procedures are indeed an effective means of accomplishing such an end.

The rational-emotive counselor serves as a live model for the client to emulate. Transference of learning, however, is facilitated when the client has the opportunity to observe other persons who similarly exhibit rational thoughts and behavior.

live models

Models in the client's real world who exhibit desirable behavior, rational thinking, and believing can be identified by the counselor, with the help of the client. The client is then encouraged by the counselor to observe these models and, in a later session, to give a thorough account of the model's behavior. The ABC method of cognitive, affective, and behavioral analysis is interwoven with the client's observations. Finally, the client is encouraged to initiate some of the model's behaviors "in vivo" — in real life.

symbolic models

Counselors, psychotherapists, and researchers have demonstrated the efficacy of symbolic modeling procedures in behavioral change (Bandura 1968; Krumboltz and Thoresen, 1964). Symbolic models are those appearing in various media as opposed to real-life models. Audio-visual media, such as films, video tapes, and audio tapes, which depict persons enacting specific desirable behaviors are examples of symbolic models. Moreover, there is sufficient evidence (Bandura, 1968; Krumboltz and Thoresen, 1964) that live and symbolic models have a greater influence on an observer's learning when the observer can identify personally and socially with the model.

In an interesting investigation (Fry, 1972), the powerful influences of social modeling on adolescent behavior have been demonstrated. Adolescent decisions regarding immediate or delayed gratification were affected by similar behaviors depicted by models in video-tape recording. Since it is often desirable to teach a client to achieve a balance in his long-range or short-range hedonistic tendencies, such results can be accomplished partially through symbolic-vicarious processes.

symbolic modeling in re counseling

Symbolic models provide vicarious observation of the behavior of others in a controlled situation and can be important to the counseling process because of the control it gives the counselor over the content and design of the experience. By reproducing a live modeling experience on film, the counselor has the opportunity to regulate and to refine the procedure. This control is especially important when it is necessary to communicate carefully and deliberately the ABC method of problem analysis. The counselor can shape more exactly what is to be modeled before the interview, thus posing a highly structured experience for the client.

The following dialogue is an example of one possible use of the symbolic modeling process in REC (through a film or video tape). The client is a young man who has just completed his education and is having difficulty in applying for a job. The example involves four different counseling sessions between the man and the counselor during which two different modeling tapes are presented. The opening interview is introductory in nature. Before he actually confronts the problem, the counselor attempts to relieve the client's uncertainties about the counseling process and explains the basic principles of rational-emotive counseling, delineating the responsibilities of both counselor and client.

The major portion of this initial interview consists of the counselor's guiding the client in articulating clearly his concern. During the session, the client expresses a fear of seeking a job and of interviewing for a job. The counselor and the client then analyze the client's problem situation. By using the ABC method, the counselor wastes little time confronting the client with his irrational ideas about the job situation. He points out that the mere search for a job is not directly causing the client's anxiety; rather, that the irrational ideas the client has ascribed to the job search are stimulating his emotional reactions. The client anxiously continues to defend his behavior and to resist the ABC method. The counselor suggests that they view a film which further illustrates the use of the ABC method. The client agrees.

In session two, the counselor introduces the film to the client, stating that it involves a young man with a similar problem and repeating that it illustrates the ABC method of problem analysis. After the counselor has answered any questions concerning the procedure, he cautions the client to be attentive to the actions displayed in the film and to relate them to his own behaviors. He then shows the film.

Modeling Tape One depicts a counselor and a client in an RE counseling session discussing the search for a job. The model counselor is extremely directive.

Counselor: You previously expressed a fear of applying for a job. Are you still anxious about this?

Client: Yes, it really scares me to even think about a job interview.

Counselor: Exactly what scares you?

Client: I get nervous because I know the job situation is very poor. It could be I'm just afraid I'm not going to get a job.

Counselor: All right; so the job situation is down, but why don't you think *you'll* get a job?

Client: After looking in the papers and talking to other guys, I can see there just don't seem to be any jobs around.

Counselor: And this keeps you from applying?

Client: I don't want to be disappointed. If I don't apply, I won't be disappointed. I know I have to look for a job, but I'm trying to delay it as long as possible.

Counselor: You think you'll be disappointed if you apply?

Client: I'll be disappointed because I won't get a job.

Counselor: You'll be disappointed because you won't get a job and you won't get a job because there aren't many jobs?

Client: Right!

Counselor: Do you mean *no one* is being hired now?

Client: Sure some people are getting jobs — the really lucky guys. I mean jobs are hard to find — few and far between. You read in the newspaper and magazines about really high-paid guys who are now having a hard time finding a job. There are a lot of experienced guys walking around out there.

Counselor: Who is getting the jobs?

Client: I don't know for sure. Some of my friends are really having a tough time too. Guys on the street have more experience than I do. I have an education, but they have a background to call upon. I would think an employer would look to experience rather than just education.

Counselor: Let's forget about all those other guys for now and talk about you. Do you think your lack of experience is keeping you from getting a job?

Client: I don't know. I don't have much experience. The competition is pretty stiff.

Counselor: Have you made any attempt to apply for a job?

Client: No. There just aren't any jobs, so why would anyone want me?

Counselor: We have spent considerable time beating around the bush and we really haven't gotten to the real source of your problem. I hear you saying lots of different things. Let's analyze your situation. By using the ABC method of problem analysis, you might be able to think more clearly about your situation. I'll diagram for you and you follow me. *(A)* represents the situation — your job seeking — and *(C)* represents your feelings — in this case your anxiety. You think *(A)* is causing *(C)*, but actually *(C)* is being influenced by *(B)* which are your beliefs about *(A)*.

Client: I don't understand what *(B)* is.

Counselor: *(B)* represents your internalized thoughts — those negative, irrational sentences you keep telling yourself. On the surface, you are blaming your fears on the job market, but in actuality, you are saying that you don't think you can compete. You may be telling yourself that you are inadequate and inexperienced and that there is no reason why anyone would want to hire you. You're afraid you'll fail — afraid you'll be disappointed. And, then, further catastrophizing, saying, "Wouldn't it be horrible if I failed?" In other words, your negative thoughts about yourself and your ability cause you to be anxious about seeking a job. Does this make sense to you?

Client: I guess so. I do feel that way sometimes.

Counselor: Now, if you are going to eliminate the anxiety you are experiencing, you will need to contradict these irrational ideas poducing it. This is where I can be of assistance to you in recognizing and altering these internalized beliefs through the ABC method. While you are here, it would be desirable for you to learn all you can about yourself. It would be in your best interest to understand the things that are happening to you at point *(B)* so you can eventually overcome the self-defeating thoughts controlling your negative emotional reactions. I know this won't be easy, but we are going to work on it together.

Following the showing of the film, the counselor and client discuss the implications of the film for the client's own situation. The client sees himself in the model's behavior. The counselor reiterates the ABC's relevance to the client's problem area. The counselor reinforces any positive thinking and behavior, and the client is given a homework assignment in which he is to practice the ABC method.

In the third session, the discussion centers on a review of Modeling Tape One. The counselor answers any questions and attempts to clear up any of the client's misunderstandings. The remainder of the session is spent rehearsing the ABC method using the model's behavior as a reference point. (It might be necessary to subject some clients to additional observation of the same modeling tape before they are able to practice efficiently the desired behavior). The client is encouraged to continue practicing the ABC method between interviews.

The counselor introduces the client to a second modeling tape in the fourth session. He explains that, in the tape, the model actually demonstrates desirable interview behavior and the successful application of the ABC method in moments of anxiety. Modeling Tape Two depicts the client who appeared in Modeling Tape One in an actual job interview. During this initial interview, the interviewer questions the model about his qualifications, interest in the job, and attitudes. He then explains the company's requirements.

Before the actual job interview, the model client practices the ABC method to combat his nervousness. As he sits in the interview, he reminds himself that it is not the job interview *(A)* which is making him nervous *(C)* but the fact that he is defining himself as an incompetent and unworthy person *(B)*.

The interview proceeds rather smoothly and the client actively engages in desirable interview behavior. He enacts the behavior well and, in general, has good control over his actions. At certain points during the interview the model begins to experience anxiety, which is indicated by nervous gestures and hesitant speech. Illustrations of his thoughts while working out his anxiety through the ABC method are dubbed into the film.

At the interviewer's mention of the need for a very special person to handle the job, the model's dubbed thoughts occur: "Wow, what does he mean by a 'special person'? There's really nothing special about me. I know I'm not the man they're looking for. Or am I? I'm really being stupid. I am really nervous *(C)*, telling myself I'm no good *(B)*, and I didn't even wait to hear exactly what he meant."

The interviewer's questioning of the model about his experience also touches off some dubbed expressions of anxiety: "That word experience again *(A)*. Why do I let it bother me *(C)*? Even though I have such limited experience, that does not make me a totally worthless person. Or, that doesn't mean I couldn't perform the job. And so I am a bit nervous — tough! *(B)*."

As the interview draws to a close, the interviewer expresses confidence in the model's potential. He informs him that several people are being considered for the position and that his name will definitely be added to the list of those considered. He promises to contact the model within a week. In his dubbed thoughts, the model responds rationally: "What if I don't get the job? I don't know if I would like to be rejected. So what if I don't get it; I'll just interview for another one. This interview has been a good experience, and it will make the next interview easier. There is no law that says things always have to turn out exactly the way I want them. I really would like the job, but if I'm not hired, I'll just try again."

Following playing the tape, the counselor asks the client to react to it. Some of the model's behaviors are practiced again. The counselor and client role-play a job interview. As a homework assignment, the client is encouraged to participate in an actual interview.

the premack principle of reinforcement in rational-emotive counseling

Rational-emotive techniques can be combined effectively with many of the standard and widely practiced behavior modification procedures, such as assertive training and social modeling. Both of these behavioral techniques are employed as a means of helping the client to achieve more effective ways of behaving. In assertive training, for instance, the counselor externally applies social reinforcement, while social modeling emphasizes self-reinforcement. Another counseling technique which stresses the client's determining or choosing his own reinforcement or rewards and, ultimately, reinforcing himself has been formulated by Premack (1965). In short, the Premack Principle suggests that a high probability behavior, such as socializing with one's friends, can serve as a reinforcer for a low probability behavior, such as studying.

Tosi, Briggs, and Morley (1971) have found that the Premack Principle serves extremely well in assisting "high-risk" college students to learn self-control over a study situation which they originally found anxiety-provoking. Essentially, in working with such students, conditions are arranged so that self-reinforcing activities follow the successful completion of a specified learning task within a given time. Both the learning tasks and the time factor are increased gradually until the college students are spending about an hour in study for each academic course. This procedure, combined with a reading skills program, has been found to influence significantly the academic achievement levels of the participants.

The use of the Premack Principle is another form of behavioral and emotional control training which is designed to help persons approach previously threatening or anxiety-provoking situations and to eliminate or reduce self-defeating emotional states. To avoid or ignore these situations might lead to negative consequences, such as expulsion from college. The use of the Premack Principle of self-reinforcement is recommended along with the ABC method of problem analysis and self-directed counseling. The idea of combining the acquisition of new behavior, self-reinforcement, and a cognitive framework in which the preceding two processes can be understood makes good therapeutic sense.

rational-emotive-assertive-training (reat)

In keeping with our concern that counselors attend to the cognitive, affective, and behavioral processes of the client inside as well as outside of the counseling session, rational-emotive-assertive training emerges as one logical problem-solving or learning strategy.

In its original form, assertive training was used by counselors and therapists to assist clients to become aware of, to explore, and to enact new and sometimes contrasting behaviors in a variety of social situations. Through a role-playing situation, the client was taught by his counselor more efficient and productive ways of expressing himself in some previously threatening social situations.

Many persons fail to assert themselves effectively in social situations because they fear some terrible consequence if they do so. Moreover, there is a tendency for some to become needlessly upset and depressed because of their failure to express themselves effectively. For instance, it is quite common for an adolescent boy to experience anxiety when approaching a girl for a date. Sometimes, the anxiety is so severe that the boy may avoid the situation and experience subsequent relief or temporary reduction in tension. The reduction in tension may serve as a reinforcer of his tendency to avoid the girl on a later occasion. In RE terms, the boy created the anxiety in himself by telling himself: "If I ask Betty for a date and she refuses me, this would be terrible. And if she refuses me, that would mean that she doesn't like me or thinks that I'm not too desirable. And since I don't know if I am that good to begin with and since I really don't compare to some of the other guys, her refusal would merely confirm my belief. I couldn't stand that." Following the act of avoiding the girl, the boy might tell himself something like this: "Damn, I don't know what is wrong with me. I must be a candy-ass. Look at those other guys who don't have any trouble at all with girls. They really have it all over me. They're something. I must be a nothing." There is little doubt that these personally evaluative sentences are associated with some rather intense feelings of worthlessness or inadequacy.

In a typical REAT session, the counselor employs a variety of techniques. Among these are social reinforcement techniques, role-playing or behavioral rehearsal, social modeling, the ABC method of emotional analysis, and systematic homework assignments. First, in a REAT session, the counselor and client jointly agree that at least one major behavioral goal will be achieved. In the case of the adolescent boy, the goal would be to increase the frequency of approaching girls for dates. Second, the counselor actively instructs the client in the ABC analysis of his self-defeating thoughts, emotions, and behavior. Third, the counselor helps the client to enact the appropriate role behavior by assuming the role of the girl. As the client successfully approaches the desired behavior, the counselor employs social reinforcement statements, such as "good" or "that's great." Prior to the role or behavior rehearsal, live or symbolic models can be introduced. Fourth, after the client's behavior has been guided by the counselor, the counselor assists the client in an ABC analysis of the role-playing situation. Fifth, the client is given a homework assignment involving an intensive study of the ABC method of problem analysis whereby the client would write out the *(As)* (events), the *(Bs)* (his self-defeating talk), and the *(Cs)* (his emotions). He is then instructed to substitute for *(B)*, a *(D)*, which would be a rational alternative. After the client has shown some proficiency in ABC analysis and role behavior, he is instructed to approach a girl with the intention of asking her for a date and concomitantly employ the ABC analysis.

In a fashion similar to strict behavioristic assertive-training, REAT places great emphasis on the acquisition of effective overt behaviors. REAT, however, augments behavioral counseling with cognitive/affective restructuring. Even though a person initiates assertive actions, he may find out for himself that there are no dire catastrophic consequences. And he may persist in asserting himself even more. Assertive behavior may replace nonassertive tendencies. The question, however, is whether or not the person has changed the negative thinking which generated his anxiety in the first place (Ellis, 1970).

Another problem associated with emphasizing only overt assertive behavior is that one of the consequences of the new behavior is social approval. While social approval is desirable, too much of it can easily reinforce a person's dire need for love and cause him even greater difficulty in the future. The indiscriminate search for approval is pernicious. It is better for the person to understand that he or she is doing the right thing for the right reasons (Ellis, 1970).

In rational-emotive-assertive training, the counselor does use social approval or social reinforcement contingent upon the client's successively approximating the desired behavior. But in the final analysis, the client learns to reinforce himself. Also, he discovers that he does not have to punish himself needlessly when he does not behave or assert himself effectively. The client learns utimately to behave effectively because such behavior is in his best interest and probably in the best interest of others. To behave solely in the best interest of others or so that others will approve of one socially is self-defeating.

new cognitive control techniques

In a 1970 address at the Institute for Rational Living in New York City, Dr. Arnold Lazarus presented six novel techniques which, when used within the broad arena of the counseling process, help reduce anxiety and bring about better individual behavioral control. Dr. Lazarus conceptualized these techniques as components fitting into the scope of a broad treatment program rather than as methods in themselves. When used as such, they augment the effects of the primary counseling procedures (i.e., cognitive/affective restructuring, assertive behavior, desensitization, etc.) and often result in the relief of tension and anxiety. Due to their emphasis of cognitive control over affective and behavioral states, these techniques readily fit into rational-emotive counseling framework.

The first technique, a means to eliminate anxiety-producing thoughts from intruding into one's daily life, is called *thought control*. This technique involves treating the obsessional thought as though it were an intruder and aggressively attacking it. This aggression takes the form of forceful inward verbalizations which are repeated over and over until the thought fades. Each individual must determine the most suitable verbalizations for himself. Dr. Lazarus suggests such terms as "get out of here" or "stop" as possible phrases.

This technique, while relatively simple, involves a certain amount of trial and error and a high degree of diligence to insure success. The following examples illustrate situations in which using the technique would be effective.

1. A pregnant woman who has previously miscarried and is plagued by fears that she will lose the second baby.
2. A teacher unable to sleep because she is concerned about a student in her class. The more she worries, the more awake she becomes.

The second technique is termed the *so what if* technique. Its focal point is people who become anxious about needless worries. When most people verbalize their anxieties, they preface their concerns with the words "what if." Two steps help these individuals to cope with their worries. The first step involves the exploration of the frequency of "what if's." This is followed by an attempt to change the individual's perceptions by having him place the word "so" in front of "what if." "What if" now becomes "so what if" and allows the individual to rationally search for alternatives to his worries.

Examples of questions where one might use this technique follow.

1. What if I don't get the job I want?
2. What if I don't make the honor roll?
3. What if I don't make the team?

The third technique, *anxiety relief* training, seems to have the same theoretical base as relaxation therapy — relaxation as opposed to anxiety. When an individual becomes involved in a fearful or tension-producing situation, he can relax himself through the repetition of certain stimulus-producing words. As do the words with the first technique, the particular words differ among individuals but must relate to calm and tranquil states. As the words ("very relaxed," "quiet," "peaceful," for example) are repeated, they become associated with the feelings of relaxation being experienced and result in some control over anxieties.

Examples of situations where anxiety relief training helps are:

1. Test anxiety
2. Fear of bugs
3. Fear of heights

The fourth technique, the *blow-up* technique, is designed for coping with anxiety in daily life. Normally, people with a particular fear avoid the fearful situation; however, avoidance only perpetuates the fear and the result is that both the fear and the tension remain. On the contrary, this technique encourages the individual to attend to the fear — to blow it out of proportion so that it becomes amusing and funny. Once the individual is able to laugh at his fears, he is ready to begin controlling them.

The blow-up technique is an alternative method to thought control. This technique is generally concerned with the fearful performance of certain acts, while thought control focuses on elimination of negative thoughts. There are, however, instances, such as the following examples, when the two techniques may be used simultaneously.

1. Fear of meeting new people
2. Fear of heights

The fifth technique, *aversive imagery*, is used for control over various kinds of compulsions, particularly overindulgence, and requires a vivid imagination as well as a strong stomach. Very often, people who are anxious tend to overindulge in various temptations. Aversive imagery, when used effectively, can become an important tool for self-control in overcoming undesirable acts. It requires the individual, for example, to imagine that the forbidden object is covered with vomit. Even as he indulges in the act, he must continue to imagine that the object is covered with vomit. Thus, as he consumes the object, he imagines he is also consuming the vomit. If the imagery becomes vivid enough, the individual will become turned off to the aversive object. The following problems lend themselves to aversive imagery.

1. Smoking
2. Eating too much

Like aversive imagery, *time projection*, the sixth technique, requires a vivid imagination. Time projection becomes useful when one is experiencing sorrow and misfortune. When an individual is distressed by the present, he imagines himself going forward in time. During this mental trip into the future, he begins to imagine all the plausible enjoyable things that could happen to him. The technique involves active sequential thinking about positive future events — first, for a day; then, a week; then, a month; etc. When the individual reaches the point where he is able to see into the future, he can look back into the past and see that there really was no justification for his anxiety. Once the individual begins to think more positively, he is encouraged to occupy his life with useful activity. Several situations are particularly helped by time projection.

1. Loss of a career position
2. Marital separation
3. Death

rational-emotive imagery

Maultsby (1972), a psychiatrist, has developed a useful therapeutic technique which he calls rational-emotive imagery (REI). REI is of considerable import because it is one of those behavioral modifying techniques which the client can apply and practice mentally outside the counseling situation and between counseling sessions.

Maultsby bases REI on the neurophysiological hypothesis that patterns of nerve impulses in the brain are the result of imagined or actual external stimuli. In general, the overall effect of real or imagined stimuli is qualitatively the same. If clients have learned traditional responses to real or imagined stimulus events, there is no reason they cannot substitute personally desirable emotional responses to such situations — even if the external event or stimulus is imagined.

Rational-emotive imagery as a counseling technique affords the client the opportunity to change self-defeating emotional states through mental practice. REI is one of the many self-teaching techniques of rational-emotive counseling. When REI is combined with real-life experiences, client learning is facilitated greatly (Maultsby, 1972). Maultsby lists three steps of REI:

1. The client is asked to write an ABCD analysis of an event or stimulus condition under which he experienced a negative emotion. (It should be recalled that the *(B)* represents irrational thinking and the *(D)* represents rational thinking.)

2. Once the client has completed the ABCD analysis, he is to decide what emotional responses he will make to the situation following rational thinking *(D)*. Then, he is to write down these chosen emotional responses and/or behaviors which follow *(D)*.

3. Once the client has mastered the rudiments of REI to his and the counselor's satisfaction, he is ready to apply the techniques outside the counseling situation. First, the client is to conjure up an image of the stimulus or situation *(A)* to which he responds with a negative emotion *(C)*. Second, he is to picture himself thinking only rational thoughts *(D)* relative to *(A)*. Third, the client is to imagine himself experiencing positive emotions to his rational thoughts at point *(D)*. The client is also encouraged to translate those imagined appropriate emotional responses to real here-and-now positive feelings.

Two cautions should be kept in mind when using REI. First, REI, like most rational-emotive techniques, is a powerful aid to behavioral and attitudinal change. Therefore, it must be used discriminately by persons who have a sufficient understanding of human behavior and sufficient training and experience in counseling. Second, if the client experiences strong negative emotional states while attempting REI and shows little progress as a result of performing such an exercise, the technique should be discouraged.

an example of rei

The client, Mrs. J, is a twenty-four-year-old black woman, married, with two children (ages seven and five). Mrs. J came to counseling in an attempt to eliminate, or at least reduce, certain marital difficulties as well as to overcome feelings of depression, apathy, and anger. She also complained of distressing physical symptoms which consisted of migraine headaches, nausea, and severe intestinal cramps. There were no apparent physical causes for these symptoms.

Mrs. J indicated that her most significant problem with her husband centered on the disciplining and caring for their children. Mrs. J felt her husband was too severe and dogmatic, placing unrealistic demands upon the children, particularly the five-year-old who has been diagnosed as being mildly retarded. For example, the husband would insist that the five year old ask her parents for permission to obtain food from the refrigerator. Later, when such demands were not obeyed, the husband responded by frequent verbal assaults on both mother and child over the child's inability to listen to and obey him. In one instance, the five year old forgot to ask permission before going to the refrigerator. When she spilled a glass of milk, the husband yelled and screamed at the child to the point that both child and mother began crying. Mrs. J typically responded to her husband's behavior toward the children by becoming violently and verbally abusive and argumentative. Every argument occurred immediately following the husband's hostile acts toward the children.

Many other interpersonal conflicts, such as relief from severe depression resulting from muscle spasms and anxiety attacks, were worked out with Mrs. J during the course of REC. Various behavioral techniques, including assertive training and systematic desensitization, were implemented. The present discussion, however, focuses upon the use of REI in the reduction of the client's volatile and angry outbursts associated with her husband's severity toward the children.

Mrs. J was first directed to identify actively the correct source of the hostility — her own irrational thinking about her husband's behavior — rather than mistakenly believing that her husband's behavior alone caused her problem. The counselor emphasized the point that it is not the action of others that truly and initially upsets or angers us; rather, it is our own view about these actions that creates the disturbance.

Mrs. J was asked to identify her thoughts about her husband immediately prior to and during the course of their arguments. With the assistance of directive and active prodding from the counselor, Mrs. J identified as her own such thoughts as:

1. "Damn it!"
2. "There he goes again!"
3. "What the hell is the matter with him?"
4. "He shouldn't act like that."
5. "Why can't I have a normal husband instead of being stuck with an idiot like him?"

At this point the therapist actively challenged the logic of the above statements. Although the first and second statements appear somewhat justifiable, they express the core of the overt hostility. The therapist suggested to Mrs. J's responses an alternate set of responses: "Nothing is the matter with *him*, although it is true his *actions* are irrational and self-defeating. Why wouldn't he behave this way — after all, this is his typical response and to state that he shouldn't perform typically is to deny reality (a sort of 'Why shouldn't it rain today?' statement). It is not a matter of why I can't have a normal husband — I simply *don't* have a well-adjusted one at present. I can choose to change this situation (either by attempting to modify my husband's behavior or seeking divorce) but until such a decision is reached, I would be better off accepting the fact that my husband is disturbed. Further, simply because he is disturbed and does stupid things, these actions do not make him an unequivocal ass. It simply reflects that his actions are often stupid and ineffectual — they are quite typical for a neurotic."

Mrs. J was given a number of homework assignments in an effort to reduce her negative emotional states. *A Guide to Rational Living* (Ellis and Harper, 1961) was suggested as an excellent supplement to the counseling encounter. Further, Mrs. J was asked to notice her hostile thoughts and challenge the reason for those thoughts and then to search for more appropriate ones. In addition, Mrs. J was required to spend five minutes each day performing REI in reference to her verbal outbursts with her husband. The REC assignment requires further elaboration. First, the assignment was issued to perform a dual purpose: to reinforce positive performance, and, more importantly, to act as a counter-conditioning technique selected to help Mrs. J acquire more suitable behavior patterns. Because Mrs. J's irrational sentences were performed with great frequency, they were habitual and were often expressed without awareness or concentration. In such situations REI is quite appropriate as a method of learning reasonable habitual responses. The method encourages reconditioning. With the aid of daily REI self-counseling interventions, one's irrational sentences and emotions are more easily identified sooner by clients.

Mrs. J's REI assignments consisted of imagining in this sequential order: watching her husband yell and scream as reinforcing one of his unrealistic demands; becoming very angry with her husband and about to yell at him; closely examining her thoughts about her husband and uprooting only irrational responses — "What the hell is the matter with him? He shouldn't yell at me like that." — and challenging such irrational ideas and then replacing them with more logical and appropriate thoughts — "There he goes again. I don't like it, but that is the way he is. That's too bad. I am going to accept this fact and also explain it to him.'"

The use of REI in Mrs. J's case confirms the theoretical rationale. Although Mrs. J did not think she could catch her thoughts in time to prevent or reduce hostility, her violent outbursts with her husband had been reduced significantly from seven a week (at least once daily) to only *one* per week after only one week of performing REI daily.

(Note: Mrs. J had been given assistance simultaneously in communication techniques with her husband. It was explained that her husband was neurotic and that the only possible method of controlling his inappropriate behavior was through an approach of understanding and acceptance).

systematic written homework

An effective method for obtaining desirable effects from the counseling setting to the client's real-life situation is that of *systematic written homework*. Written homework further provides an excellent vehicle for coordinating cognitive, affective, and behavioral processes in an individual and thus facilitating positive growth to an optimal level. Developed by Dr. M. Maultsby (1971), the technique consists primarily of assigning to the client the task of analyzing emotional states through the ABC model in writing.

The writing assignment is structured according to a typical ABCD paradigm. *(A)* is the actual event or happening; *(B)* is the person's thoughts about *(A)* (self-talk); *(C)* is a description of the emotional responses or feelings; and *(D)* is alternative thoughts to *(A)* (rational-alternative self-talk). *(D)* is divided into two distinct processes. First, the client analyzes the *(A)* section to determine if it is an accurate description of objective reality. This analysis is followed immediately with a sentence-by-sentence challenge of the *(B)* section in order to correct any illogical or inappropriate thinking.

An example of a typical written homework assignment more vividly illustrates the format. The client is a seventeen-year-old student in high school who has difficulty in academic performance compounded by an "interpersonal conflict" with one of his teachers. A typical homework excerpt follows:

A. *Facts and Events*

"I was called upon by the teacher to respond to a question when it was obvious I didn't know the answer. When I failed to respond the teacher made fun of me in front of the whole class."

B. *Thoughts*

1. "That Bitch!"
2. "She knows I don't know the answer but she just wants to put me down."
3. "Why the hell should she call on me when I can't answer?"
4. "I am not going to do a damn bit of work for her."

C. *Emotion:* Intense Anger

D. *Alternative Thoughts*

1. "She is acting bitchy but that doesn't make her a bitch. Although her behavior is anything less than perfect at this instant, that does not mean that she is at all times a worthless slob."
2. "She might think that I don't know the answer, but she can't be sure since she can't read minds. Also, it may be true that she wants to put me down but I can't know that for sure. It is only a guess."
3. "Why shouldn't she call on me? It would be nice if she didn't, but the fact remains that she did, and for me to deny or try to change what already has happened will only result in future discomfort for me."
4. "Discomfort not for her but for me. Not doing my work hurts me in the long run, not her."

The use of SWH by clients offers many advantages, among which are transference of counseling gains to real-life settings and the co-ordinating of cognitive, affective, and behavioral processes. In addition, written homework will assist in combatting the law of inertia which alludes to man's inability to get started in initiating change. Often, clients enter counseling with a long history of irrational thinking; sometimes, they have reached a point where the irrational behavior is habitual. In such cases, mere reflection and concentration may have limited therapeutic value. Written homework, however, if applied consistently, may provide needed impetus in the production of desired change.

Ellis has devised an objective means to assess one's performance outside of the counseling session. The homework report format attends to the client's emotional states, his actions, and his related beliefs or thoughts. The instrument is quite valuable in that it permits the client to assess his own self-defeating and irrational cognitions, emotions, and behavior as well as determining for himself or at least attending to self-enhancing and rational self-processes. (See Homework Report on page 83.)

systematic desensitization and relaxation training in rec

Wolpe (1966) has devised an approach to psychotherapy which he has called *systematic desensitization*. The effectiveness of this behavioristic psychotherapy has been demonstrated with clients who suffer from severe anxiety. In essence, the technique involves three operations: training in deep muscular relaxation; the construction of anxiety hierarchies; and counterposing relaxation and anxiety-producing stimuli contained in the hierarchies.

In systematic desensitization the client is first taught to relax himself thoroughly. Secondly, when relaxation has been achieved successfully, the client is asked to imagine scenes which depict anxiety-producing events which have been ordered on a continuum ranging from least anxiety-producing to most anxiety-producing. The underlying idea is that if a strong antagonistic response (relaxation) to anxiety is made to occur in the presence of those stimuli which induce the response, it ultimately will inhibit the anxiety response. Thus, the client will eventually come to associate a relaxed state with situations that were previously associated with a state of anxiety. Systematic desensitization proceeds initially with the least anxiety-producing stimulus being paired with relaxation.

HOMEWORK REPORT[1]

Consultation Center

Institute for Advanced Study in Rational Psychotherapy

45 East 65th Street, New York, N.Y. 10021 / (212) LEhigh 5-0822

Name ———————— Date ———————— Phone ————————

Instructions: Please draw a circle around the number in front of those feelings listed in the first column that troubled you most during the period since your last therapy session. Then, in the second column, indicate the amount of work you did on each circled item; and, in the third column, the results of the work you did.

	Amount of Work Done			Results of Work		
	Much	Some	Little or None	Good	Fair	Poor

Undesirable Emotional Feelings

1a Anger or great irritibility	1b	___	___	___	1c	___	___	___
2a Anxiety, severe worry, or fear	2b	___	___	___	2c	___	___	___
3a Boredom or dullness	3b	___	___	___	3c	___	___	___
4a Failure to achieve	4b	___	___	___	4c	___	___	___
5a Frustration	5b	___	___	___	5c	___	___	___
6a Guilt or self-condemnation	6b	___	___	___	6c	___	___	___
7a Hopelessness or depression	7b	___	___	___	7c	___	___	___
8a Great loneliness	8b	___	___	___	8c	___	___	___
9a Helplessness	9b	___	___	___	9c	___	___	___

[1] Albert Ellis, "Homework Report" (New York: Institute for Advanced Study in Psychotherapy). Reprinted by permission of the author.

83

HOMEWORK REPORT (continued)

	Amount of Work Done			Results of Work		
	Much	Some	Little or None	Good	Fair	Poor
10a Self-pity	10b			10c		
11a Uncontrollability	11b			11c		
12a Worthlessness or inferiority	12b			12c		
13a Other (specify)_____	13b			13c		

Undesirable Actions or Habits

	Much	Some	Little or None	Good	Fair	Poor
14a Avoiding responsibility	14b			14c		
15a Acting unfairly to others	15b			15c		
16a Being late to appointments	16b			16c		
17a Being undisciplined	17b			17c		
18a Demanding attention	18b			18c		
19a Physically attacking others	19b			19c		
20a Putting off important things	20b			20c		
21a Telling people off harshly	21b			21c		
22a Whining or crying	22b			22c		
23a Withdrawing from activity	23b			23c		
24a Overdrinking of alcohol	24b			24c		
25a Overeating	25b			25c		
26a Oversleeping	26b			26c		
27a Undersleeping	27b			27c		
28a Oversmoking	28b			28c		

84

	Amount of Work Done				Results of Work		
Undesirable Actions or Habits	Much	Some	Little or None		Good	Fair	Poor
29a Taking too many drugs or pills	29b ___	___	___	29c	___	___	___
30a Other (specify) _____	30b ___	___	___	30c	___	___	___
_____	___	___	___		___	___	___
_____	___	___	___		___	___	___
Irrational Ideas or Philosophies							
31a People must love or approve of me	31b ___	___	___	31c	___	___	___
32a Making mistakes is terrible	32b ___	___	___	32c	___	___	___
33a People should be condemned for their wrongdoings	33b ___	___	___	33c	___	___	___
34a It's terrible when things go wrong	34b ___	___	___	34c	___	___	___
35a My emotions can't be controlled	35b ___	___	___	35c	___	___	___
36a Threatening situations have to keep me terribly worried	36b ___	___	___	36c	___	___	___
37a Self-discipline is too hard to achieve	37b ___	___	___	37c	___	___	___
38a Bad effects of my childhood still have to control my life	38b ___	___	___	38c	___	___	___
39a I can't stand the way certain people act	39b ___	___	___	39c	___	___	___
40a Other (specify) _____	40b ___	___	___	40c	___	___	___
_____	___	___	___		___	___	___
_____	___	___	___		___	___	___

PLEASE PRINT! BE BRIEF AND LEGIBLE!
ANSWER QUESTION C FIRST;
THEN ANSWER THE OTHER QUESTIONS.

A. Activating event you recently experienced about which you became upset or disturbed (Examples: "I went for a job interview." "My
mate screamed at me.")

_____

_____

rB. Rational belief or idea you had about this activating event. (Examples:
"It would be unfortunate if I were rejected for the job." "How
annoying to have my mate scream at me!")

_____

_____

iB. Irrational belief or idea you had about this activating event. (Examples:
"It would be catastrophic if I were rejected for the job; I would
be pretty worthless as a person." "I can't stand my mate's screaming; she is horrible for screaming at me!")

C. Consequences of your irrational belief *(iB)* about the activating event
listed in Question A. State here the one most disturbing emotion,
behavior, or consequence you experienced recently. (Examples:
"I was anxious." "I was hostile." "I had stomach pains.")

_____

_____

D. Disputing, questioning, or challenging you can use to change your irrational belief *(iB)*. Examples: "Why can't I stand my mate's screaming and why is she horrible for screaming at me?")

_____

_____

cE. Cognitive effect or answer you obtained from disputing your irrational
belief *(iB)*. (Examples: "It would not be catastrophic, but merely

unfortunate, if I were rejected for the job; my giving a poor interview would not make me a worthless person." "Although I'll never
like my mate's screaming, I can stand it; he or she is not horrible
but merely a fallible person for screaming.")

_____

_____

bE. Behavioral effect or result of your disputing your irrational belief *(iB)*.
(Examples: "I felt less anxious." "I felt less hostile to my mate."
"My stomach pains vanished.")

_____

_____

F. If you did not challenge your irrational belief *(iB)*, why did you not?

_____

_____

G. Activities you would most like to stop that you are now doing:

_____

_____

H. Activities you would most like to start that you are not doing:

_____

_____

I. Emotions and ideas you would most like to change:

_____

_____

J. Specific homework assignment(s) given by your therapist, your group, or yourself:

_____

_____

K. What did you actually do to carry out the assignment(s)?

_____

_____

L. Check the item which describes how much you have worked at your last homework assignment(s):

     _____ a. almost every day

     _____ b. several times a week

     _____ c. occasionally

     _____ d. hardly ever

M. How many times in the past week have you specifically worked at changing and disputing your irrational beliefs *(iBs)?*

_____

N. What other things have you specifically done to change your beliefs and your disturbed emotional consequences?

_____

_____

O. Check the item which describes how much reading you have done of the material on rational-emotive therapy:

     _____ a. a considerable amount

     _____ b. a moderate amount

     _____ c. little or none

P. Things you would now like to discuss most with your therapist or group:

_____

_____

_____

_____

Although rational-emotive theory embraces most of the systematic desensitization procedure, it disagrees with its highly mechanistic-deterministic position which places the person at the mercy of external stimulation rather than his own internal stimulation. In short, the *(B)* or the cognitive component of the ABC paradigm is deemphasized in desensitization. Therefore, when systematic desensitization procedures are called for, I combine them with some of the REC procedures.

One critical component of the desensitization procedure is the client's ability to engage in emotive imagery. The assumption is that cognitive symbolic representation of real stimulus conditions is possible for eliciting affective responses. It would seem that the mere images of anxiety-producing situations, in and of themselves, produce anxiety. In reality, however, another cognitive process, such as labeling, probably moderates emotive imagery associations. For instance, a person will ascribe verbal labels or other symbols to those external events which have taken on anxiety-producing properties. That is, he labels, defines, and evaluates those events in such a way as to minimize or maximize their anxiety-producing effects. Rational-emotive theory would hold that the cognitive interpretive-evaluative process, the one that the person himself engages in is the one most directly associated with his anxiety.

RE counseling makes use of desensitization techniques but clearly augments those techniques with ABC analysis. While teaching a client to relax himself thoroughly and then counterposing relaxation with graded aversive stimuli on the anxiety hierarchy (desensitization), the therapist also teaches his client new and more effective ways of achieving greater cognitive control over his emotions.

Relaxation training is a physical means of inducing positive emotional states. Such a procedure can be combined with other techniques aimed at associating appropriate thoughts and sentences with relaxed states as one progresses along the anxiety hierarchy. I have found that one useful procedure during relaxation training is to pair certain rational sentences with those differentially induced states of tension and relaxation. I have used this technique in group counseling with young married couples and have found it to be quite successful in achieving self-control over anxiety reactions associated with intimate contact between hubands and wives. The following relaxation procedures were first applied in such cases:

1. Tense muscle in specified area.
2. Observe muscle tension in specified area (about ten seconds).
3. Notice difference between muscle tension and other sensations.
4. Maintain tension for about thirty seconds.
5. Gradually reduce tension.
6. Continue relaxation (focus on relaxed state for about ten seconds).

Muscle relaxation of the following parts of the body was taught to each group participant:

1. Right arm
2. Left arm
3. Lower right leg
4. Lower left leg
5. Right and left feet
6. Forehead
7. Jaw
8. Tongue
9. Eyes
10. Neck
11. Shoulder
12. Back
13. Abdomen
14. Right and left thighs

The client also is encouraged to practice relaxation exercises about thirty minutes each day. Relaxation training is complete when the client can arrive at a state of relaxation without applying the tension exercises first.

When there is evidence that the client can discriminate between tension and relaxation states during training and focus his attention on these differential states, the counselor can intermittently introduce the following ideas or cognitions:

1. Under conditions of muscle tension: "Relative to the scene you are imagining, what you experience is tension; it is painful and uncomfortable, but it is not a terrible or horrible feeling."

2. Under conditions of muscle relaxation: "What you are experiencing is a state of relaxation which is a more comfortable state than is tension relative to the scene you are imagining."

the use of tape-listening in rec

In the initial stages of counseling (awareness, exploration, commitment), the use of *tape-listening* is an efficient technique for helping clients master these stages. The use of tape-listening (Maultsby, 1970) permits the client to experience self-induced positive reinforcement for his involvement in the counseling process. Moreover, as an audio aid, it forces the client to focus upon his irrational thoughts, emotions, and behavior within the interpersonal-therapeutic context. As a technique, it was designed to induce the client to evaluate and appraise himself in accordance with RE theory, and, specifically, in terms of the three criteria for rational thinking.

The technique (Maultsby, 1970) of tape-recorded listening consists of the following steps:

1. Record all counseling sessions.
2. The first five taped sessions are saved permanently. (If important critical incidents have occurred in other sessions, those tapes are also saved).
3. Either between twelve and seventy-two hours following a counseling session or twelve hours before the next session, the client is scheduled (under the counselor's supervision) to listen to his tape as often as he can. In so doing, the client is asked to apply ABC analysis to his behavior during the counseling session.
4. If a client is highly upset at the end of a session, he is encouraged to listen to the tape-recorded session immediately.
5. When clients demonstrate significant growth as a result of their counseling experience, they are scheduled for an additional listening session each week. This is done until the client has had a chance to compare the latter session with each of the first five sessions.
6. About six weeks before the counseling sessions terminate, the routine is repeated again. (In short-term RE counseling, this sixth step may be unnecessary).

In counseling situations where a client is unusually resistant, I have been able to reduce his resistance by having him listen to the tape of the session immediately. In such cases, I spend the first half hour of the session counseling the client and the second half hour supervising his tape.

five * rational-emotive counseling and encounters

This chapter places in operation in counseling practice the parameters presented in Chapter One, the philosophy and concepts of REC described in Chapter Two, the expression of client irrational thinking presented in Chapter Three, and the use of some of the RE techniques discussed in Chapter Four.

The verbatim counselor-client interchanges in this section were all based upon my own cases. There is one exception, the verbatim role-playing session "To Abort or Not to Abort," which was contributed by Dr. W. A. Carlson, a former teacher and colleague of mine. A number of issues facing our youth are presently here; although the cases are not completely representative of all issues on the youth front, I do believe, however, that the more critical psycho-social processes underlying human behavior are evident in the encounters that follow.

Some of the more significant personal issues and concerns are expressed here by persons trying to discover themselves and involve love and intimacy, identity, sex and guilt, and self-acceptance. I also believe that the sessions portray the work of therapists and counselors who quite actively, directively, and sometimes forcefully intervene in the lives of their clients.

Because our theoretical models only approximate reality, the counselor-client transactions here are far from a perfect fit into the theoretical structures that guide the efforts of counselors. As you follow carefully these exchanges, you will not observe a one-to-one correspondence between theory and practice. But you probably will notice that RE interventions are indeed quite appropriate and powerful means of dislodging ideas that are largely responsible for a person's emotional and behavioral disturbances.

stages of the counseling process: towards a greater capacity for love and intimacy

One characteristic of the healthy person is his capacity to love and be intimate with others. Today, our youth particularly seem to place a high priority on the importance of interpersonal intimacy, loving, and caring. Few people in our society have a reasonable definition of love as well as the capacity to affirm a sensible definition. As a counselor works with his clients on matters of love and intimacy, he encourages them to develop and affirm a personal and self-enhancing definition of love.

In *The Art of Loving* (1956), Eric Fromm presents a brilliant analysis of love. He addresses himself to the neurotic and the self-defeating notions of love as well as to the more reasonable and self-enhancing meanings of love. Fromm explores *counterfeit love, romantic love,* and *mature love.* Counterfeit here is depicted as an expression of certain underlying self-defeating tendencies such as masochism and sadism. Romantic love involves the person's projection of ideas into the other whereby he ascribes to that other person certain characteristics which emanate from his own emotional needs. Mature love is an outgrowth of a process in which a person has transcended the stage of romantic love and/or neurotic love. It is characterized by a union of two persons who are able to affirm their individual identities and integrity. Again, the capacity to love maturely depends largely upon one's basic trust in himself — a belief in his ability to be himself in spite of others and a belief that he can survive and grow personally alone or with another person.

In adolescence, love often symbolizes an attempt by a person to affirm his identity. He does this by projecting into the love object his own self-image in order to test it, explore it, and to clarify it. The self-image or concept, it will be recalled, involves a complex set of cognitive, affective, and behavioral processes. In short, one's self-image is that which a person believes about himself at a given moment. On the matter of loving another person, if one's self-image is based upon an irrational set of beliefs, he will tend to project that irrational image onto others. On the other hand, when one's self-image has evolved from a basic sense of trust and a reasonable philosophy of life, such a sense will characterize his projections.

Through a variety of social exchanges, an individual may determine for himself whether or not someone fits his projected ideal. One reason people are attracted to one another is that they attempt to mutually validate their beliefs and attitudes by seeking agreement from one another. As a person tests his projected ideals in an interpersonal context, he does so by indicating to himself the new information arising out of the particular social interaction and then tries to find confirmation for his system of beliefs. In social exchanges between men and women, for instance, there will be greater attraction if they hold similar beliefs and attitudes toward various symbols. But if the meanings, beliefs, or attitudes toward the same set of symbols are irrational in nature, the attraction may be of a self-defeating variety.

The human act of love or intimacy is rooted in the belief-value constructions of the person. In essence, the person, as he interacts with another person, indicates that other to himself, defines and appraises the other, judges the other, selects features to respond to, and organizes himself to act. Therefore, much of what is observed in interpersonal interaction and attraction is self-interaction. In specific rational-emotive terms, when a person's personal meaning about objects or symbols is of an irrational or distorted nature, it is difficult, if not impossible, for him to become intimate with another person or to express a genuine love. The process by which a person indicates to himself another person and ultimately responds to that person will largely be a function of how reasonably and realistically he defines and appraises himself and that person.

In summary, persons project onto other persons certain unfulfilled needs which take the form of idealized fictions. The ideal is the possibility of fulfillment, and these projections are, in some cases, developmentally unhealthy or neurotic. The counselor's task, then, becomes one of assisting his client to become more cognizant of the differences among the types of love, to accept and understand these differences as they relate to him, and, ultimately, to affirm his own definition of love which eventually may lead him to a happier life.

The following dialogues are excerpts which illustrate the stages of the counseling process as these stages relate to one issue — irrational ideas about love. The issue of love and intimacy was extracted here to provide some operational meaning for the stages of counseling. In actuality, other problems, such as excessive drug usage, relationship with parents, and difficulties in holding a job, were confronted in these counseling sessions. The client was a young man of twenty-three years of age.

the awareness stage

Client: While I was living with my girl, I couldn't stand the bitch. . . . She was on my ass all the time. . . . She tried to change me. . . . All that nice shit she whipped on me, "But I love you, and I want the best for you," and, "I want you to love me and you don't act like you do." . . . Damn, she pissed me off. . . .

Counselor: You mean that you didn't like the way she acted.

Client: No shit. Let me finish. OK?

Counselor: Sorry, go ahead.

Client: Now I am all fucked over. I started to run around with other chicks and my chick kicked me out. . . . Now I want her back and she won't hear me. . . . She doesn't want nothing to do with me. . . . Man, I didn't realize how much I love her.

Counselor: *(At this point, the counselor does not reinforce the client's ideas about love. Instead, he places a different label on the feelings expressed by the client. The counselor, however, does not tell the client that he is not in love.)* You mean, you now realize that you now need her. Is that correct?

Client: Yes!

Counselor: That's bullshit. *(Counselor challenges the client.)*

Client: What do you mean?

Counselor: I am not too sure about your beliefs or the definitions you have about love, but I am reasonably sure that while you may desire your girlfriend for one reason or another, that is not the same as having a dire need for her or saying to yourself, "I need her or I can't survive." *(At this point, the counselor approaches the client's belief system or those internalized sentences about his girlfriend which are the real sources of his disturbances.)*

The counseling session continues in about the same vein. As the counselor confronts and challenges the client's irrational beliefs about love, it is crucial for the client to see that much of his emotional reaction is the result of how he appraises his situation and then ascribes a value to it — good or bad. The counselor introduces the client to one of the most basic ideas of rational-emotive theory: That negative emotions are biased, prejudiced, and irrational evaluations and appraisals. Obviously, the client is not totally aware of the counselor's strategy. But the counselor does not keep his strategy a secret for very long. Specifically, the ABC method of problem analysis is introduced by the counselor.

Counselor: Let's see if this type of analysis makes some sense to you. At this point *(A)*, there is your ex-girlfriend. Let's for the moment consider her an external event. Now at point *(B)*, you tell yourself something like this: "I realize that I still love and need her and it is terrible that I can't have her." At point *(C)*, you experience a feeling of anger or "pissed" OK.

Client: That's about right.

Counselor: It is somewhat interesting that you blame your girlfriend at point *(A)* for your anger and depression at point *(C)* when, in fact, it is the nonsense you're telling yourself at point *(B)* which is the most direct cause of your feelings, namely that is awful or terrible that this girl should reject . . . Moreover, you are probably saying rather grandiosely "that she doesn't have the right to do this to me, after all I've done for that bitch." Right?

Client: No.

Counselor: And even at a deeper level, you are probably telling yourself that "I must be an incompetent idiot for not being able to win her back. And, after all, am I not a worthless shit anyhow?"

Client: Well. I don't know about all that.

Counselor: OK. Let's back up a bit. I can understand that you might feel badly when you strongly desire something and can't have it.

Client: OK.

Counselor: But that's one thing. It is another thing to tell yourself that "it is terrible that she isn't doing what I want her to do and I can't stand it." What's so terrible about that?

Client: She makes me feel bad.

Counselor: No, you make yourself feel bad because you are not getting exactly what you want from her. And you are making matters worse by saying that she should or ought to take you back and because she should, it is terrible that she doesn't.

Client: Well, I guess.

Counselor: And I even would guess that you go on and say to yourself that "since I really and truly love her because I have these strong desires I should not be rejected because that hurts me even more, and, therefore, she should take me back because her rejection causes me to feel miserable." Not only is this thinking highly confusing and illogical, it is the reason why you are disturbed. And it is one reason that it would be in your best interest to reassess and redefine some of your thinking and believing about love and intimacy.

Before the counselor and client terminated the first counseling session, the counselor explicated the ABC method of problem analysis to the client, instructed the client in the use of the technique relative to his thoughts and emotions about his girlfriend and prescribed two reading assignments — selected chapters in *A Guide to Rational Living* (Ellis and Harper, 1961) and *The Art of Loving* (Fromm, 1966). In the awareness stage, it is essential that the client acquire a cognitive framework to facilitate his self-understanding and his participation in the counseling process.

The client eased into the exploration stage after about the second session. Into the third session, he started to relate himself more fully to the new information gathered from the readings and the homework assignments.

the exploration stage

Client: I read Fromm's book on loving as well as selected chapters in the Ellis book.

Counselor: Did these readings, along with what we talked about, make any sense to you?

Client: Well, some.

Counselor: Tell me.

Client: It makes some sense. Especially the chapter on dire needs for love and approval. I'm not sure whether I go along with the idea that no person really needs another person. People need people. I guess I need the girl.

Counselor: Would you die without her?

Client: No. But I would be unhappy.

Counselor: You mean you would be as you are now — depressed.

Client: I guess. I don't know.

Counselor: OK. Not having her is not to your liking. It would be nice to have her now. It would be nice to have her hold you, caress you, and even ball you wildly and passionately. But since you don't have her — and, I admit, it might be nice — what in the hell is so terrible about it?

Client: Because, goddammit, I have to have her.

Counselor: You mean you have to have her body or her loving attention, her sexuality, all of the pleasurable things she gives you. Is that right?

Client: No.

Counselor: Look, you had all of that before, didn't you? And you also had all the shit she gave you along with that. Now, that's what you couldn't stand — her shit. So you left. Now you have forgotten that and can remember only the good things.

Client: Maybe it will work this time.

Counselor: Maybe it will. Maybe it won't. What's the difference?

Client: Well, if I have these dire needs for love and approval and that's why I am depressed because I'm not getting exactly what I want upon demand, maybe if that is so and I work that out, I would be happier.

Counselor: Well, that is probably correct.

Client: Maybe my girl will even take me back.

Counselor: Yes, maybe. No, maybe. What would be so terrible if she didn't?

Client: You know I think I am confused about love. Really confused.

Counselor: OK. Maybe you are. What's so bad about that? As a matter of fact, isn't that one reason why you are here?

Within the exploration stage of the counseling process, the client is to relate himself, in his present thinking, feeling, and behaving, to new and possibly more self-enhancing ways of functioning. Exploration, as are other stages, is self and situational in nature. The counselor persists in confronting and challenging actively the client's irrational ideas and beliefs about love by posing a contradictory position. The idea is to help the client modify his irrational thoughts *(B)* about his girlfriend *(A)*. In spite of the client's resistance to the counselor's efforts, the counselor keeps hammering away at the client's resistance but accepting fully the client's right to resist. In this particular interchange, the client showed increased hostility towards the counselor. The counselor simply accepted the client's right to be hostile, but, later on in the session, pointed out to the client that his feelings of depression were in part the result of his internalizing hostility. It was shown further that excessive externalization or internalization of hostility can be self-defeating, even though some of it is natural. Furthermore, following hostile acts, there is the great tendency on the part of humans to condemn themselves further, to become even more depressed, and to sustain such feelings over a long time. The ABC method of problem analysis and confrontation was employed by the counselor to help the client make sense out of his feelings. The client also was given a homework assignment in which he had to apply the ABC method to his problem situation. In other words, he had to put his new ideas. to the empirical test. Thus, it can be said that reality testing is central to exploration.

the commitment stage

The client's commitment to his own effective personal development was evident in about the fifth session. Commitment, it will be recalled, is an outgrowth of awareness and exploration.

Client:　　　I have given a great deal of thought to the things we have talked about in here. *The Guide to Rational Living* has been useful too. I have tried practicing and working on those homework assignments . . . You know, the ABCs. I think some of that stuff is beginning to work. I don't feel as depressed as I did before.

Counselor:　Good. How about Paula?

Client:　　　Yeah, Paula. Maybe I have been making heavy demands on her — expecting her to kiss my ass and all that, but, goddam, I still have those terrible fucked-up feelings about her. I know they're fucked-up, but I still feel them. I really feel like I got to have her back.

Counselor:　OK. That's where you are. I know that you're confused, but in your confusion, that's bad.

Client:　　　It's bad, but I guess, in your words, not catastrophic. Look, Dr. Tosi, I haven't been that successful in applying that ABC analysis.

Counselor:　So what. It is not necessary that you become an expert overnight.

Client:　　　Well, all I know is that I probably have a ways to go, but I'll keep working. Can I really get over this shit?

Counselor:　Yeah, if you work your ass off.

the skill development stage

Skill development does begin in the early sessions, but it is not a salient phenomenon until later in the counseling. The client's entry into this stage was noticed in about the sixth or seventh session.

Client:　　　I've finally reached the point where I've finally gotten the idea of this ABC analysis. You know, I've been able to get myself feeling a lot better about my situation with my ex-girl. As a matter of fact, I am practicing this method almost daily. It works more effectively. I used to become disturbed about little things, but I can see the potential.

Counselor:　Good!

Client:　　　It feels good. Before I really believed that my life almost depended on my girlfriend taking me back. I blamed her for my feelings. Now I can finally see that I have been disturbing myself all along the way.

Counselor:　I understand that there are things that you liked about your girl and still like. But I had a hard time with some of your personal definitions of love and intimacy, especially some of your self-defeating, grandiose, and impossible demands you introduce to those concepts.

Client: I am beginning to reevaluate those definitions, and, you know, when I do that, it puts myself right into what I am all about. At times it amazes me that I am capable of projecting a lot of my shit into other people. I am doing that less.

Counselor: That's good. Now let's be a little more specific about how you are developing these attitudinal and behavioral modifying skills.

The session continues, and the counselor listens attentively to the client's explication of the ABC method in light of his problematic situation. During this time, the counselor makes sure the client is effectively replacing his irrational ideas with more rational ones. He and the client also discuss further behavioral change strategies for *implementation* and *practice.*

Within a three-to-four week period, the client, with the counselor's active intervention, was able to develop the ABC skill in analyzing and reconstructing his ideas about love and intimacy. It was just a matter of time before he refined this skill (skill refinement).

the redirection, change stage

Though client growth is observed through the counseling session, at the final stage, one can observe the client's cognitive, affective, and behavioral processes occurring in a more unitary fashion. He now has a greater capacity to redirect himself through these stages at a higher level and in relation to other matters of personal concern. The client manifests a greater sense of cognitive control over his emotions and behavior, and because he no longer needs to deceive himself, he is by definition a more authentic person who is capable of choosing and thinking for himself.

Counselor: How have you been these days? Or, more specifically, what has your thinking, feeling, and behaving been about your ex-girlfriend?

Client: Simple. I think I've finally accepted the fact that we probably won't get together again. But, that's OK. I really don't need her. As a matter of fact, I was really kidding myself all along. I feel cleaner, I guess. You know, I have been sexually involved with some other girl in the last four weeks. For the first time, I didn't have to prove myself as a man; I honestly enjoyed sex. I even told her a lot about what I've been through with you in these sessions. I don't know if she understood, but I did make an attempt to let her know where I am.

Counselor: That's good; you're relating much better with girls.
Client: Yes and I'm able to understand them better. Sometimes that's scary, isn't it?
Counselor: Maybe so. But whatever the case may be, one's growth and and development don't have to stop. The crucial factor is that you have to engage in and expand the same kinds of processes you engage in here throughout your life and in a variety of situations. As a matter of fact, on this love and intimacy matter, you will probably be developing and growing for a long time, but I think you have finally captured an important process.

george c.: lead us not into temptation

George C. decided to enter individual counseling when he became emotionally upset over his marriage and his own sexuality. George C., a student in counseling and psychotherapy, is twenty-five years old and has been married for about seven years. He and his wife have three small children aged six, four, and two. George was married immediately after high-school graduation. He entered college and majored in history and education. During his college years, he became associated with a jazz-rock group and decided to "go on the road" with the band. He was an unusually talented musician, and within a short time gained some national recognition.

Upon finishing undergraduate school, he continued to work as a musician for about three years. Financially, he was successful. About a year ago, George C. decided to enter graduate school and pursue a major in counseling and guidance. He was considered by the faculty to be a bright, dedicated student with much potential. His major interest was in the area of humanistic psychotherapy. He was exposed to rational-emotive therapy through independent study and courses in counseling practicum.

When George C. entered the counseling situation, he knew ahead of time what to expect from it. He was aware of my orientation and had observed several of my demonstrations. Because of this, I wasted virtually no time with the usual relationship-building strategies with George. For this reason, I felt very secure about confronting him with what I believed to be some core issues during the initial session. At the outset, I assumed an extremely active and directive posture.

Since George was aware of RE counseling and had explored it for himself in his own practicum, I did not explain the principles of REC, such as the ABC or homework techniques, during the first session. Instead, I merely included them as a routine part of the counseling process.

George initiated the session by stating that he needed attention (reinforcement) from women to build his "ego." He complained about feelings of anxiety and guilt over the thought of his wife discovering him in having extramarital relations. In this first session, I tried to show George how he was defeating his own ends. This session focused primarily on a rational-emotive analysis of guilt or self-deprecation. Moreover, the client was confronted forcefully with his refusal to take the constructive actions needed to contradict and overcome his emotional disturbance. Toward the end of the session, George was given some homework assignments designed to initiate ABCD self-confrontation of his negative emotional states. Following the actual session, I also asked for some of George's personal reactions to the counseling session.

interview

Client: It's my ego. I have a terrible thing with women left over. I mean I keep needing reinforcement. You know what I mean?

Counselor: With chicks?

Client: Yeah. And there's no way to reconcile it cause I'm married so I can't go out and test it and if I do, I get really guilty. So it bugs me wondering why I have to keep needing this. I know that it's just ego, if that's what you want to call it.

Counselor: That's a good word.

Client: Yeah, but that doesn't help. Like a couple of years ago, I'd go running around, but I wouldn't get into bed, I'd always come up with an excuse. Like I just wanted to see if I could get there. Then that didn't help because then I'd tell myself that anybody could get there. So that didn't help either. So I keep going around in circles.

Counselor: Yes, and no matter what you do, you can't fill up that thing you call ego.

Client: Right.

Counselor: But you still have it and you still want to fill it up.

Client: Right.

Counselor: Well, can you describe it a little more?

Client: Yes. Well, I get a number of variables in there, reasons for why I'm doing this. Like I have an ugly thing going. Like I'm convinced I really got ugly in the last few years. When I first came down here, there were chicks all over me. In high school, I wasn't any big flash, but I didn't have any real problems. But then down here when I let the hair grow and got into some music, chicks came easy, but I knew it was the image attracting them, not me. Then I got married real young, and we went through the usual crap of hating one week, loving the next. Then I accused her of getting lax; she'd accuse me of running around which I wasn't, so then I did. She knows that. I don't know. I just still have this sex thing. I like chicks. But if I try to get it together, I can't. If I do, I have this real guilt thing.

Counselor: OK, two things. You like chicks; that's one thing. The thought of chicks is pleasing to you.

Client: Yeah, but it's base 'cause it's all sex.

Counselor: What do you mean it's base?

Client: Well, it's not like I want to go have some nice meaningful relationship with someone.

Counselor: Yeah, you just want to fuck.

Client: Yeah, like my wife is great. But when she's not around, like when I'm walking down campus, I just go nuts.

Counselor: Okay, so when your wife's around, things are okay; it's just when she's not around.

Client: No, it's worse when she's not around 'cause I get more daring.

Counselor: Well, if she isn't around it gives you the opportunity to check some of these chicks out. OK. On one level, you say, "Look, I want to go out and fuck." And you say that's base. Now I don't hear that completely because on the other hand you're saying it's ego too.

Client: When I said base, I didn't mean in a moralistic sense, I just meant that all there was was the sex.

Counselor: What I thought you were saying was this: "Look, I just want to fuck for the sake of fucking; it has nothing to do with ego or anything else." But then a little while ago, you were saying it's ego too. How much of it is just basic raw sex on your part?

Client: It's fucking for my ego is what it is. They're both there.

Counselor: OK, so the two overlap. So you sit around at night thinking, "Well, my wife's gone now and since I like to fuck so much, now would be a good time to get out and look around. But, what a shit I would be, especially if I actually got hold of some babe and fucked her."

Client: Yeah, but I worked that one out too. I'd only feel guilty if I get caught or 'cause I was afraid I'd get caught.

Counselor: OK. Right. So it's if she found out this would be a terrible thing. What would be so terrible if she did find out?

Client: She'd kill me.

Counselor: She would? She wouldn't shoot you, would she?

Client: No. OK, it's like this. I've figured out the antecedents to why I do this. Like sometimes I sit around and resent the fact that I got married so early and missed these things.

Counselor: OK, you've got what I would call insight number one.

Client: Right. Then, you know, we had a baby right away and I've been tied to the house since I'm seventeen years old. Then, for the first few years, I was working with a jazz group, and there were thousands of sexual opportunities which I passed up and I'd see all these other guys, married, not giving a shit, fucking their brains out. Then my wife and I had had some bad times, not talking and everything, so I went out, once, got laid, and got the clap. No justice. And I told my wife about it. I didn't have to 'cause we hadn't made love in quite a while, but I got guilty and told her. Man, I have never felt like such a shit in my whole life. She was a wreck, but she came out of it and was really understanding. But she made it very clear that if it ever happened again, I go out the door.

Counselor: So, in other words, you say, "I don't know about getting the clap again, but if I go get laid, she could not handle this horrible thing; she would blow her mind, and as a result of her becoming needlessly upset and disturbed, she would leave me and I would be out in the cold."

Client: Yeah. But OK, like now, our relationship is very good and most of the time when I'm home, I can forget it. But I don't know . . . yeah, I do. OK, like I don't feel as attractive as I used to and that's why I need that support from the outside. . . .

Counselor: OK. Let's check that one out. *(A)* you like to fuck, let's say that's a biological given; *(B)* you're also saying you need to fuck for your ego because you don't feel as if you have as much shit going for you as you used to. Is that close to what you're saying?

Client: Yeah, but I always pretty much controlled the fucking scene either 'cause I was afraid of getting caught or something, but just finding out I could get there was enough.

Counselor: OK, as it's like this. You gotta go check out how much shit you've got together with chicks. It's submitting your ego, which seems to be a rather grandiose ego, to the empirical test. Is that about right?

Client: *(Laughs).*

Counselor: It is kind of funny, but it seems somewhat true.

Client: Grandiose . . . that's right.

Counselor: But it almost appears as if you're saying, "Look. I really don't have an ego and I'm trying to get one."

Client: I don't know; I never approached it that way; I just assumed I had one.

Counselor: Well, you do have one. OK, let's take the subject of your own sexuality. You say, "I've got to prove that I am someone desirable to other people, especially women; I need the reinforcement. When I get the reinforcement, that proves that I am a reasonably healthy, functioning male."

Client: I don't know.

Counselor: Let's check it out.

Client: I have no question of my functionality. It's one of these both wanting and not wanting to be married scenes. See I've got it separated in my mind, on my side, between sex and marriage. At the same time, if she went out on me, I couldn't handle that one either. So I do this resentment thing. You know, like I'm married but do I have to be dead? Like eveybody I know is always out fucking around. But I don't want to get into a blaming thing either. It's like I love my wife very much and want to stay with her but at the same time, I find marriage very restrictive. I think she resents it if I go out with my friends, and she doesn't have any girl friends she likes going out with so. . .

Counselor: OK, here's what I'm hearing. You say, "She lays a lot of shit on me and if I don't come around to her way of thinking, she'll get pissed off, and I don't want to hurt her so I'll give in, but then again, I don't want to give in; I want to define my situation a little differently than she's defining it for me.

Client: I'm not really sure I've got a line on where all this started. When I was playing in the jazz group, she resented me playing. She had valid reasons. Like she was home all the time and I was out playing. But she blamed the whole thing on sex. You know, all the girls that follow bands around. Now I don't know if it was really that or just the fact that I spent more time on music than her that got her pissed or jealous. Then, that pissed me off and that's when our hassles started. She began laying accusations on me and I wasn't fucking around but then I began to. I don't know if it started with the sex thing or if she talked me into it. Maybe it was because now I'm spending a lot of time at the school, and she doesn't hassle me as much. She hassles, but it's more subtle and she does it through the kid.

Counselor: That's more legitimate, but, OK, let's say your wife has some problems. Maybe she's afraid that you'll go out and run around and withdraw your love from her. She gets very upset and acts in a very controlling manner as a result of that. Now, that's her problem and we can talk about her all day. I'm beginning to get a feel for that situation. Now, you tell me, "Look, I've got to prove myself," let's say, through other women or with other women sexually "for my own ego." Now, that's your problem. So that may or may not have a whole hell of a lot to do with your wife, although the two are related.

Client: In one specific area. See when we got married, my wife really freaked me out; she was gorgeous. Then, after the baby, she kind of let go and she's never gotten back, and that's like seven years. So physically she's just not as attractive.

Counselor: See, I hear this ego thing. In other words, I need someone who can space me out, who's physically attractive. I really do; that's what I want because when I have that, I feel good. Why did she do that horrible thing to me?

Client: Sure, I like that.

Counselor: Right. I can understand that. What you're saying is that after the kid came she withdrew herself, especially her physical self from me.

Client: I don't see it as the kid versus me or anything. I just kind of resent her letting herself go. And if I say something about it, she uses it for an excuse and says she doesn't feel attractive so I ask her why she doesn't work at it and we go in this circle.

Counselor: So you feel powerless. As if you want her to come through for you in certain ways and she says, "Look, I can't pull it off; there must be something wrong with me," and you say, "Shit, I don't have any influence."

Client: Yeah, well I feel sort of semirejected by that. At first, I'm not so sure anymore; it might have been an excuse I was using, but I'd think, "Well she thinks she's got me hooked and she doesn't have to do anything anymore." That I resented and that's when I started looking at other chicks.

Counselor: In other words, "My wife isn't treating me the way I want to be treated." OK? And because she isn't, I can't stand it. And goddammit, there's no one in this world that's going to get away with that shit for long. I'll show her, or someone, or myself that I am quite capable of being felt as a man or person or as anything. And, by God, I'll show her that I've still got a lot of spark left in me. In other words, since I always did like chicks (which is kind of normal for anybody, but in your case I think you're beating

	yourself over the head with it), I'll go out and show her that I am something highly desirable."
Client:	No, I don't want to show her.
Counselor:	OK, here's the thing. You may not want to go out and say, "OK, honey, watch me; now, here I am." But in your own head, you probably do that symbolically. Understand? You're chasing broads down the street, and one of them gives you the come-on. Whether or not you go with her you're saying, "Hey, man, I could make it with her, and that proves unquestionably that I'm a he-man of some type. But I've also got some real questions about that." Is that about right?
Client:	Yeah. But I'm not sure, uh, I think if I really tried, I could.
Counselor:	Right. If you walked down the street this minute and asked ten broads to go to bed with you maybe three or four would say yes right on the spot. Maybe they would tell you to get lost. Who knows?
Client:	No, I don't know about that. All right, let me give you a concrete example. I went to a bar this weekend with a friend, and by the time the night was over, I had five pieces of paper in my pocket from chicks, which I later threw away. Like I wanted to go, but I got paranoid. Maybe if I would've gotten drunk enough, that would have given me an excuse.
Counselor:	OK, you've got the papers and you're pretty sure the chicks will screw, but, again, you raise the question, "Well, if I do this and my wife finds out about this, wouldn't it be terrible because then she'll come down on me even more?" Is that about right?
Client:	Yeah. But it's not her coming down on me; it's her splitting. I don't want to lose her.
Counselor:	That's what I mean. You don't want to lose her, but you're not totally happy with her behavior towards you. In other words, you're saying, "I need more than what she's ready to give me at this point, for my own ego. But if I go out and get that, it would be horrible if she found out and I couldn't live with the guilt. But then, in another sense, I enjoy and relish the thought of doing it."
Client:	That's right except for one thing. It's not her. I'm not putting blame on her.
Counselor:	Right. That's extremely reasonable.
Client:	See, I realize that my demands are unreasonable. I think I'd pull this with anybody. You know, goddammit, like everybody else is going out so I am too.

Counselor: OK, so you know that. You know that she's got problems, but just because of that, it doesn't mean that you have to have problems.

Client: Right. She's not the cause of my problems.

Counselor: OK, so then what the fuck are you telling yourself?

Client: I tell myself a number of things. Like its unreasonable to have to limit myself to one chick sexually.

Counselor: Yeah, and its also highly unreasonable and horrible for you to do so.

Client: Then I tell myself it's unreasonable to risk a good relationship just to get my rocks off. I go back and forth between these things. Then I bring in others around me and think, "Look at that fool, fucking every night of the week and he gets no shit." I think a lot of this guilt shit is just 'cause I got the clap. Like I felt condemned, you know, one time, wham.

Counselor: Like out of the clear blue sky, God came down . . .

Client: and ripped me off. No, really, that's true. This is all a part of my mass confusion about existence. I spend all kinds of time looking for a reason. I've done incantations to God, to the devil, to the sea, you name it, looking for a reason behind all this.

Counselor: Well, probably the reason is that you went out and got laid and the chick was clapped up. It's as simple as that.

Client: Yeah but . . .

Counselor: You're looking for some kind of mystical-magical explanation.

Client: Yeah. I sit there and say what kind of shit is this? I stay clean for years and then . . . Like I never even balled another chick the whole time we dated. Like I was in bed hundreds of times and then copped out of screwing because I knew the guilt would be coming. So that's like six years all together. Then I go out once and get zapped while everybody I know is screwing constantly and nothing.

Counselor: OK, so what's deterring you from screwing?

Client: Getting caught.

Counselor: Getting caught, then condemning yourself. "Poor wretched me. All those other bastards are getting away with it and look at me. Look at all the shit I get. Poor me." Isn't that about it? Poor me.

Client: Yeah, I do that.

Counselor: So we're back to this same thing, poor me. "OK, I've got some things going for me, but in some areas, I'm really deficient. So I've got to go out and demonstrate to people that I'm something desirable." That's what I hear you saying.

	I also hear you saying if you don't prove to yourself that you are capable, that would be a horrible thing. And I'm saying, what would be so horrible if you never went out and proved yourself sexually or otherwise?
Client:	Well, when you started talking about that, I did this. See, I generalize this whole thing; it's not just related to sex or marriage. See, I'm never in the middle, I'm always on an extreme. Like intellectually, I either visualize myself as a complete moron or as a genius. I never see myself as just a normal guy. I do this with everything.
Counselor:	What I hear you saying is this: "I've got to have a whole lot of shit going for me, otherwise I have nothing. If I'm not number one, I might as well be the shit I think I am anyway." Now that kind of thinking can only get you into a hole. Is that what you're doing?
Client:	It's not a competitive thing.
Counselor:	What do you mean, competitive?
Client:	With anybody else.
Counselor:	All right; it might just be that in your head you're saying, "I've got to be number one with me, at all costs." Such thinking is just as pernicious.
Client:	Yeah, I compete with myself.
Counselor:	Yeah, "I've got to be number one in everything because if I'm not, I might as well be the total shit I tend to think I am anyway. That's why I have to be number one." Does that make sense?
Client	No, if I get some little satisfactions along the way, I'm all right. But I guess it's all the crap I have to wade through to get there.
Counselor:	And I don't want to wade through all the goddamned crap.
Client:	Yeah. And, also, I have nothing that I believe in completely, that I won't compromise on. Then if I do, I feel like a shit for giving in. Like my job; I hate my fucking job. But I want the money. I see the job as useless, myself useless in the job; I resent the job being stupid. I resent myself being stupid in the job. I feel used by the job and that I'm using it.
Counselor:	Yeah, well, with that kind of thinking you lose every fucking time.
Client:	Right.
Counselor:	So you've applied that same logical sequence to your sexuality, your masculinity, your ability as a student, your work; so what else is new? Now you're coming in here telling me that you've got a big fucking ego, when you're really saying, "Look, I'm not too sure what the hell I'm all about. And that's terrible and that's horrible." I raise the question:

What's so horrible about you being confused at this point in your life? Or even being somewhat disturbed about your own confusion? What's so horrible? I'll tell you what's so irrational about it — because I got to be perfect. I may not be competing with someone else, but I've got to be something other that what I am. And since I'm not that which I want to be, I must be something less than desirable. And hence I'm going out spinning my damn wheels trying to prove it here and there ad infinitum. And even if I do prove it and I'm successful 100 percent of the time, I gotta worry about keeping it up." Is that right?

Client: Yeah, but I know all that. I know I set things up so I can't win and go in circles.

Counselor: OK, you know it, so the question is: How do you stop it? That's the therapeutic question. "How do I stop this endless putting myself down?" See, it seems to me that you've got a pretty good idea of how you got where you are. We call that insight number one in REC, knowledge of the antecedents that initiated your nutty thinking. Being a student of counseling and psychology yourself you probably have a thorough knowledge of psycho-dynamics. Insight number two is that you have a pretty good idea of what you're telling yourself to disturb yourself. In other words, you have an idea about what those screwed-up thoughts of yours are and how those thoughts are causing your screwed-up feelings. So you have two types of insights and that's nice, but there's a third type that you may need to acquire and ultimately accept, and that insight is that if you're going to change your philosophies you will have to work and practice. In other words, you will need to learn to contradict that bullshit you're telling yourself, cognitively as well as behaviorally. Now, you haven't come to grips with how you are going to initiate constructive actions outside of counseling. But the thing you're going to have to learn is to deindoctrinate yourself literally. That is, to challenge and to contradict your stupid fucked-up thinking. For example, how do you know that you're a shit? And even if you convince yourself of it, what is so goddamned terrible about being a louse or a goddamned incompetent fool? Anything? If you could prove it in the first place.

Client: Yeah, it doesn't meet what I want to be.

Counselor: OK, that's true and you might be annoyed at that fact.

Client: Yeah, but the reason I can't work this out knowing what I do is that the condemnation half of this comes from other people.

Counselor: You may have originally gotten some ideas from other people.

Client: No, I mean it's in relation to other people. Like if I go out, I don't feel guilty for me; I feel guilty for her . . .

Counselor: Now that's bullshit. If you're feeling guilty, you're feeling guilty because you're beating yourself over the head for one reason or another. You're trying to change the reasons around for why you feel guilty. If you didn't feel guilty, how would you possibly feel guilty about someone else? You might be concerned about them or you might feel somewhat badly but you wouldn't be needlessly disturbed. See, you're saying, "I don't feel guilty if I go out and fuck, but I feel guilty to think that my wife would find out and she would leave me and this would be horrible and she would define me as a shit and in her eyes I would be a shit and I don't really think I'm a shit." That's what you're saying and that doesn't make any sense. The fact of the matter is you're probably telling yourself, "If she finds out that I went out, she would condemn me, and I couldn't stand being condemned so I'll go on condemning myself for not wanting to be condemned by someone else." That makes more sense than what you originally said.

Client: I guess that's right.

Counselor: You guess that's right. Are you tuned into what I'm saying or not?

Client: Yeah.

Counselor: Yeah? Then tell me what I just said.

Client: I can't be guilty for someone else; I'm guilty for me regardless of what directions I try to pretend it's coming from.

Counselor: Yeah, and don't bullshit yourself about it. You're literally beating yourself over the head with it. Probably what's happening is this: "I don't like myself for having to go around proving my worth through external kinds of achievements such as going out chalking up fucks." Let's get it sorted out. Does that make sense?

Client: Yeah.

Counselor: Yeah what?

Client: I know what you're saying.

Counselor: OK, good; now, what are you going to do about it? That's the crucial question.

Client: The problem is that when I'm not engaging in those guilt-producing activities, I feel like I'm wasting away. Like why am I sitting on my ass watching TV? And if I do, the guilt is so intense it makes it not worth it. So I sit and maybe two years later when the guilt mellows down, I'll do it again.

But my mind has so much more power than my body, it's ridiculous; I can just drive myself crazy.

Counselor: Well, that's probably accurate. It's kind of like what you're doing now. Convincing yourself that you ought to be disturbed because you're not getting your fucking way about things. That's probably it. See you pose impossible situations for yourself. You come in here and you know you've got insights number one and number two; you know you're disturbing yourself; you're in touch with a lot of this shit, but you're still disturbed.

Client: Yeah, 'cause I don't see a way out.

Counselor: There's only one way out and that's to begin to challenge the bullshit you're telling yourself. You've been around me long enough to know there are ways to contradict what you're telling yourself. You know that. What you are saying is "Yeah but I can be so lazy, and so tired, and I just don't have the energy to get off my fucking ass and do something about it." Which, by the way, is one of your damned major problems. In an existential sense, you think a lot about coming to grips with things but refuse to do a damn thing about them. You come in here and lay out fifteen different things: Wife, ego identity, who knows, but you still have a hard time doing anything with your knowledge about them. It's easier for you to sit on your ass than it would be to face up to your own growth, development, sanity, or whatever you want to call it.

Client: OK. But when I work these things through, I'm still nowhere, like on the sex thing, I'll think, "OK, asshole, if you do it you're guilty; if you don't, you're horny so you lose both ways so all you can do is stop being a fucking baby and forget it and stop it."

Counselor: Right and stop it automatically, immediately because really coming to terms with it would involve a hell of a lot of work. So instead you're going to grandiosely will it to come to an end, never really confronting the major problem.

Client: Yeah that's what I do because it stops and it works for a while, but then it's back again.

Counselor: OK. The fact of the matter is that you might have urges to go out and screw; you even think about it. But you're saying it's catastrophic just to think about this kind of thing.

Client: Only because I get pissed off that I can't.

Counselor: That's right; you don't get your way, and that's horrible. So thinking about it is one thing; actually doing it is another thing and beating yourself over the head about it is still another thing and actually the most pernicious goddamned thing you can do. When you beat yourself over the head, you literally reindoctrinate yourself with that insane shit that makes you feel like a nothing; then you want to go on to prove that you're a something. So you perpetuate a vicious cycle and then you go on to wonder why you feel shitty about yourself. But you know why you feel shitty about yourself? Because you have insights one and two, but you won't get off your ass to do something about your problems and "What a shit I must be for not working on them." See!

Client: Yeah. The only action I ever contemplated besides like you said automatically stopping is suicide.

Counselor: In other words, I'll really be grandiose and end it all and show all these bastards and they'll all be sorry or something.

Client: No that's never entered it.

Counselor: All right.

Client: As a matter of fact, my wife and I argued about this once. She knew I was thinking about it and accused me of being selfish.

Counselor: Maybe she's right on that. If not selfish at least grandiose.

Client: I guess.

Counselor: Look, the fact of the matter is that you were goddamned fucked up; at that point you said, "Look, I have to solve the problem and I don't know how, but there's one way that solves it forever." The only problem with that, from an existential point of view, is that it then negates, or denies, or wipes out any other possibility. At least, if you stay fucked up, the possibility of later getting it worked out is there. You see what I mean? Your problem is a very simple one. You're having a hard time with the law of inertia. You know what that is. It has to do with people who have problems and also have a hard time getting started in solving them. It's much simpler to lay back because then you never have to test yourself out. Interestingly enough, if you begin to contradict some of the bullshit you're telling yourself, you have made a good start tackling the law of inertia.

Client: If it works.

Counselor: Yeah. If it doesn't, so what? See, in your case, if it doesn't work in two weeks, then you've demonstrated to yourself that you're incapable and incompetent. The fact of the matter is that if you're going to grow you will have to do one goddamned thing and that's to get off your ass, even if it takes twenty goddamned years. Otherwise you've got a lifetime of misery. Understand? Now one of the reasons you're here after not talking to too many people about this is that you've decided that it's time to tackle some of this shit. Now I want to help you do that. We have to get one thing straight. Your number one problem is inertia. You're having a hard time getting off your ass and engaging in what we would call constructive action in a cognitive and behavioral respect. So now, if you're going to move and expedite this whole process, you will need to translate your ideas into actual practice.

Client: Yeah, I know it. I have to do some thinking about tackling this.

Counselor: Yeah. As a matter of fact, rather than just thinking about it, you want to begin to think in terms of some things you already know and begin to put these things into practice. As a matter of fact, I'll give you some papers on the subject written by Dr. Maultsby that you can read for yourself. Do you have any other reactions or comments?

Client: I'm wondering how it's to be done. This has been going on for so long. It gets better and worse. There are times when I'm bugged by something and no matter what I do, I can't get rid of the awareness of it.

Counselor: That's not unusual by the way. As a matter of fact, You are quite good at maintaining the things you're telling yourself that get you disturbed. Like "I'm a wretched no good shit and I've got to prove to the fucking world and myself that that I've got something going for myself. Even though I've made tremendous gains that's not enough. I've got to be some superhuman."

Client: But sometimes I turn that around and say, "I'm so fucking great that it makes no sense that I have to suffer all this other shit. Who has the right to get in my way." But then I say, "Who the fuck are you to demand that?"

Counselor: Right, you come down on yourself; that's the point I was trying to make. OK, what we'll do is begin to tackle these concerns of yours in more reasonable ways. The idea is for you to learn the therapeutic techniques that you've been studying to apply to yourself. Understand?

Client: Yeah. That's the bitch; I study these things and say, "OK, that works," but you come out a robot.

Counselor: OK, there's the bullshit. You say fine, but grandiosely add, "How does this apply to *me*?" The fact of the matter is that if you begin to work, take some of these ideas you've learned and apply them to yourself day in and day out and really make a commitment, yeah, they'll work. Or you can sit back, reading and writing and studying about this shit, and never applying it. Then you'll stay right where you are.

Client: That's where I get hung up. I read this shit and think it really looks like it works, but I get stuck between the metaphysical thing and the rational thing. It's much easier for me to throw the rational thing at people I'm working with than to put it on myself. Then I can't figure out how they use it and get happy.

Counselor: Well, they're probably taking your expert advice and really practicing. What you're saying is that you have a hard time applying to yourself the knowledge you have. What I see is a basic existential concern getting in the way — that is action.

Client: Well, I don't see existential people as happy.

Counselor: That's bullshit. Some existentialists are miserable like some atheists are miserables, etc. What the fuck else is new?

Client: I guess what I'm saying is that all this has to do with convincing yourself.

Counselor: It's making a commitment really. In your case, making a commitment to get off your ass and apply some of the ideas you've learned about human growth and development. You have insights number one and two from an REC point of view, but you're having a hell of a time with insight number three which has to do with commitment to work, work, work, (i.e., applying the ABCD analysis). That's where we have to go. Fortunately, as a result of your training program you're involved in, you're learning many new things and there are interested people around here that can help you grow, but we're not going to sit around and reinforce the shit you give us. You really wouldn't want us to. Would you? Well, it's interesting that you're pretty much in tune with the ways we operate and that's nice because it does help to expedite the counseling process. I don't have to explain as much. Let me give you a few handouts; here is a personal homework report developed at the Institute for Rational Living by Dr. Ellis. It will help you work on your concerns in a more systematic way. Fill this out for me this week. It really involves ABCD analysis of problems and emotional disturbances. So come back the same time next week and we'll talk about your reactions to the homework and also pick up where we left off today. OK!

crisis counseling:
to abort or not to abort

a role-playing encounter with dr. william a. carlson

In this session, Dr. William A. Carlson demonstrates crisis counseling in which he works with an unmarried, pregnant girl of twenty-one years of age. The session depicts a soft RE counseling style which is direct and active but highly expressive of empathy and understanding. This is a decision-making session. The decision "to abort or not to abort" is one of the major concerns of many young women today. It reflects an important contemporary issue, one a counselor functioning in any setting has encountered or will encounter. In usual RE fashion, Dr. Carlson, in assisting the client in making her decision, not only emphasizes and accepts the client's self-induced anxiety and guilt, but, at the same time, also tries to help her eliminate those self-defeating emotions which are associated with her concern.

Although the counseling session which follows is a role-playing session, it is very realistic. Following the session, the client did express strong feelings of anger and anxiety about the problem which she talked about. She had been able to make it, at least temporarily, very much part of herself. The counselor felt the same way about the counseling session, as did the advanced students in counseling and psychotherapy who observed the session. All of the ten students in the class, some of whom were doctoral students, believed that the session was, in fact, a live counseling session with a client who really had the problem which she stated she had.

Counselor: I think as you know I'm Dr. Carlson and you're Pat. What do you prefer as your calling name?

Client: Pat.

Counselor: As you know and as you can see, there is a TV camera here. There are possibly other counselors. This is being taped on TV and also on audio. Now, what is taped on this is confidential with the counselors here in this center. OK?

Client: Yeah, I guess that doesn't really matter. It might make me a little nervous but it's not like anyone is going to be talking about this to somebody.

Counselor: That's right.

Client: OK. Sure.

Counselor: Now, I understand that you called to come into counseling, that you wanted to see me. What understanding do you have in terms of counseling?

Client: Well, what it is, I've got like this decision to make and thinking it out myself, I just can't do it. I don't know what I want to do and I just thought I needed someone to help me, help me make it. Maybe the way I'm thinking about it — maybe I'm too wrapped up in it — to see it in a clear way. I just know that by myself I'm not able to do it. I thought that maybe by coming in and talking about it — well, you can't make it for me — but maybe you can show me where I'm not thinking straight. I'm just at this point

	where I don't know how to make it and need help in making a decision.
Counselor:	It certainly sounds like you're feeling a heck of a lot of pressure here.
Client:	Well, what it is, a couple of months ago I thought I was pregnant and I kept putting it off and I found out last week that I am. I don't know what to do. I don't want the baby; I really don't, and I'm not going to get married for sure. And I don't want the baby. I'm just scared to death of having an abortion. And that's it. I've got to decide — I don't want this kid, and I don't want to go through childbirth. I'm not straight on abortion yet; I still feel like I'm taking a life. And there it is.
Counselor:	Now, let me try to understand this a little better, Pat. How are you so sure you are pregnant?
Client:	I went and had the test at the Health Center — it came out positive. It has been two months that I've missed my period.
Counselor:	By medical examination, you're two months pregnant. And did the physician talk to you about the difficulty in this situation?
Client:	No, not really. I just got the results. Then I came out last week and went home and told my roommate. We've been talking about it. She thinks I ought to have an abortion because I don't want to marry. Since it just happened a week ago, I haven't told him yet. I just wanted to be able to make a decision because I don't want to hassle him because there is no reason why he should have to be in a hassle. I've just been like really upset this week and my roommate is the only person I've told and like I said, I couldn't come to a decision by myself, and the only thing I could think of was professional help. I've got to decide whether I'm going to have the abortion or the kid, I guess.
Counselor:	It seems like you're trying all sides of this. Like at one point you're saying, "I couldn't possibly give birth" . . .
Client:	Oh, God, I really don't want to.
Counselor:	. . . and on the other side, you can't convince yourself that you want to go on the abortion route because you feel you are taking a life.
Client:	It's like both options I don't want to take. I have to take one of them — I don't see a third. So that's where I am. I try to think myself into one or the other and just get . . .
Counselor:	Let me just kind of back up for a moment. What has your thinking been on being pregnant? What has this meant for you?
Client:	Since I found out?
Counselor:	Well, before and now.

Client: Yeah; before, it was something I never thought about in connection with me. Pregnancy is something that happens to other people. I could never have thought of myself getting pregnant, being a mother. I guess it's sort of denial that it could happen and when it hit, it was just like everything dropped — it was like my world dropped; "My God, look what's happening, you're going to have a baby." My feelings right now are "Why did this have to happen?" It's like I feel bitter.

Counselor: Bitter in what way?

Client: Like why do I have to go through this thing?

Counselor: In a sense is this a matter of being angry?

Client: Yeah, I'm angry that it had to happen and I guess it's my fault too because we weren't real careful. I wasn't on the pill — I had this thing that I didn't want to go on the pill. And what we were using — we weren't always careful (foam and rubbers); we didn't use them all the time. Like if it is this far away from the middle of the month, I guess it's OK not to be using them, but I guess it wasn't OK.

Counselor: Is it maybe anger with yourself or anger with him?

Client: Yeah, it's a little bit of that too although I see I shouldn't be angry with him.

Counselor: Is there maybe something else going on here; what about feelings of guilt?

Client: I don't think I feel so much guilt in having sexual relations really; I'm just mad at myself that I was so stupid not to realize and take the proper precautions. I mean, if that's what you're getting at, I don't think I feel guilty.

Counselor You're saying that you understand all of this, that you knew what to do, even thought of getting the pill and somehow managed not to. How did you do that?

Client: About the pill — I didn't do that because I was afraid of gaining weight and there are some slight effects that come with certain people, and I thought that the protection we were using (foam and rubbers together) was as effective as the pill but that I only had to use those for the middle ten days. It's just like during those other days, "Well, I can't get pregnant now." Because I was really regular so I felt for sure there was no way. I just told myself that it was just a few days ago, and we don't have to use them.

Counselor: And so from everything you can sense within yourself right now, there was nothing of guilt or upset about the sexual part.

Client: No, I think I worked that out quite a while ago.

Counselor: Apparently, then, one of the big things that came up was a lot of anger, principally at yourself for misjudging.

Client: Like "Oh boy, we did it now." That's how I feel.

Counselor: Now where does that come from — getting so tough on yourself?

Client: That I should have known better. I should have known that you can't take chances. Now I know it; you can't. The doctor told me when I went for my pelvic: Use foam and rubbers all the time, but somehow I talked myself into only having to use them for those ten middle days.

Counselor: And now you're dragging on the fact, "Oh, God, I should have used them all the time."

Client: Oh, God, I sure should have or I should have gone on the pill even.

Counselor: Now, look, this for a major part is a lot of feelings of anger that you should have been more safe.

Client: Well, I should have.

Counselor: Well, in a sense it would have been a good idea, but there is no law which says you absolutely have to and obviously there wasn't a thing to do. Interestingly, what happens is what really should have happened.

Client: It had a chance of happening anyway.

Counselor: With everything set exactly the way it turned out, the results are precisely what should have happened. What sense is it to keep thinking to yourself that it should have been different?

Client: I guess none. I guess we just have to accept that it happened.

Counselor: And yet is there a kind of feeling of sadness there? You say to yourself, "OK, there is the way everything is run; no one could expect possibly the results which happened but it did."

Client: But at the time I didn't expect it; I thought it wouldn't happen.

Counselor: In a sense, there is no magical way to just go back to the pregnancy itself. You thought about that I bet though.

Client: Sometimes I would like to do things and think things like "It's not true." Like I'd wake up and it wouldn't be true.

Counselor: Then you'd open your eyes a couple more times and know it was true.

Client: True; I did that a lot before I was really sure.

Counselor: Since the doctor said you are, it's becoming more of a reality to you.

Client: It's just like a constant weight on me.

Counselor: You've been torn between the two feelings and you've been switching. You have to come to help and understand the

	original ideas and feelings of anger, how do they seem to you now?
Client:	*(Pause.)* I'm still angry with myself for not having taken the precautions I should have, but it's overshadowed now by a desperation to get something done, to get the thing settled. I've got to come to this decision because it's just eating me up.
Counselor:	Well, let's look at what the possible alternatives are which you laid out pretty clear when you first came in — birth or abortion — which one should we talk about first?
Client:	Giving birth — WOW — that's another thing in pregnancy I can't imagine myself doing. I don't want to do it; I really don't.
Counselor:	It seems to me that the main feeling, the main ideas that come to you when you think, "OK, here I am pregnant, and if I don't take steps, I will have to give birth." What's the meaning of this to you?
Client:	Complete disruption of my life forever, well at least six months or more; disruption that I can't finish school — after one semester, I'll have to be out; the hassle of my parents finding out which they would if I gave birth. I'll have to give the baby up; I don't want the baby — readjusting after I have it. It seems like things have been going so well and now here this thing is and for the next six months, I'm going to have all these problems. One main one would be telling my parents, I just — WOW — they wouldn't take it at all.
Counselor:	So giving birth to the child would not only disrupt your life in terms of time span and prevent you from doing all the things you really have planned but also in terms of telling your mom and dad.
Client:	Yeah, they'd just be upset — sure. They'd really be upset.
Counselor:	What would your parents think?
Client:	Well, for one thing, the idea that I'm having sexual relations. I've talked the things over with my father — when I even mention that I condone it in others, he really gets upset. He said to me, "I know, Patty, you'd never do something like that; you couldn't face us if you did." I just let him think it.
Counselor:	What was the message you were hearing there?
Client:	Darling daughter, you could never do that . . .
Counselor:	And you don't dare.
Client:	Oh sure, yeah, absolutely. So I just let him think it — that I was an angel.
Counselor:	Are they pretty generally easily upset over sex or over any sort of thing?

Client: They both get upset easily over little things; yeah, they do, but that's just a flare-up. But this is something that's really ingrained in them from what I can tell; from talking to them about others and how they react about other people who have sex before marriage or who have to get married. It's really a strong point with them.

Counselor: Even letting them know anything about this, they're really going to blow.

Client: I really feel that way.

Counselor: Now, are there any other feelings or ideas that come to mind when you think of giving birth?

Client: That I don't want to go through with it; it's painful; I'm really afraid of it.

Counselor: Look at the other side of it now — the abortion, your feelings and ideas about that.

Client: See, that's what I want to do because it gets rid of the problem. The only thing I have is that thing that I'm still not settled that I'm not killing a life. As much as I hate that life for being there, I just have that . . .

Counselor: Now, here again, I hear anger.

Client: Yeah, I guess I was angry. I'm angry. I almost said I want to kill it.

Counselor: Has the thought entered your mind, not leaning towards it, but leaning towards yourself?

Client: Slightly, every once in a while — killing myself would end the problem — but not real seriously.

Counselor: Have you ever sat down and planned it?

Client: No, not at all just that, "I should kill myself."

Counselor: Why not?

Client: 'Cause I don't want to kill myself.

Counselor: That really surprised you for a moment when I asked you that. It disturbed you, didn't it?

Client: Yeah, it kind of surprised me.

Counselor: Now what does your answer tell us?

Client: That I do want to live.

Counselor: So those are only momentary thoughts, almost like the magic solution to this all. You are creating the anger. How do you manage to be so angry?

Client: Because it's like ruining my life right now; it's making me miserable.

Counselor: OK, in a sense it's giving you a little pain in the ass. You certainly wish it were over now. You wish you would have taken the doctor's advice. The anger — how are you creating the anger?

Client: *(Pause.)* It goes back to myself; I'm saying, "You dumb ass, look what you've gotten yourself into." I look at it; the anger I guess is at myself because I have no logical reason being angry with it. I did it; it didn't have anything to do with it.

Counselor: Now, how are you being able to be angry with you?

Client: *(Pause.)* Because I'm telling myself, "You got yourself into almost the worst situation you could get yourself into right now."

Counselor: Well, in a sense it probably is true; you did get yourself into a lousy situation, but how about the anger, how are you angry with yourself?

Client: I think probably because I haven't made a decision. It's like I'm being forced to make a decision I don't want to make. It's like I get so angry at this thing being in me and like I've got to make a decision one way or the other, and I don't want to do it; I don't want to do either of them.

Counselor: So, apparently, you feel that your hands are being forced into one lousy decision or another lousy decision and that the whole world ought not be that way.

Client: I shouldn't have to do this. *Yeah, like I'm damn angry that it happened, that I have to — shit — yeah, that I have to do this.*

Counselor: Now can you see this, Pat, that this could be why you are angry, that you're in a situation whether you like it or not; you're forced into a decision, a decision which will be made even if you do nothing about it.

Client: That's right.

Counselor: And that you can build yourself up with all kinds of demands that you ought not be pregnant, you ought not have to make the decision; it sounds like what's been bothering you.

Client: Yeah, that's what I've been doing. When I get angry I think, "This shouldn't have happened to me."

Counselor: Now turn it the other way around and begin to find a solution to "I shouldn't be in this jam; it shouldn't have happened to me; I shouldn't have got pregnant; I shouldn't have to be facing this decision;" then comes the anger. Does that make the feeling for you?

Client: Yeah, that's when I get angry, when I think about it.

Counselor: Now what can you do to take away the anger? Or maybe we should go gack to the prior question: "What would it mean not to be angry even if you're in this jam?"

Client: Well, if taking away the anger is going to help me make a decision, then that's what I want.

Counselor: Do you think the probability is pretty good that if you felt less angry then it would be easier to decide which way to go?

Client: Yeah, because being upset is really making me — when I think about it, I get really upset.

Counselor: You're going around in a circle and not doing anything about it. And the anger — I think we're essentially in an agreement here and you're the one who has to answer "yes" or "no"; that there is the demand that it shouldn't really be but really is.

Client: *(Pause.)* By accepting what I don't want to accept — it happened and I have to accept it.

Counselor: Like it or not, you're pregnant and . . .

Client: *(Outburst.)* BUT I DON'T LIKE IT . . .

Counselor: And nobody said you have to like it. Now, how does this sound; how does it fit?

Client: It still gives me a twinge to say it: "I'm pregnant." It still does. I think maybe I haven't accepted it fully. I guess I wouldn't until I really start showing it, feeling it, then I'd really . . .

Counselor: Well, more real in the sense of reality. It's just that realistically you have a problem and one way or the other it will be solved, and that you still have time, some chance to participate in the decision.

Client: I'm not so sure that I have that realization of the child in me.

Counselor: In one sense, particularly if you go on making the decision, maybe you won't want to. Now, come back and see the alternatives that you laid out very early today in the session — to give birth or abort. What types of ideas do you have on this now?

Client: It's like right now I really want an abortion; it's like if I can have the abortion with no guilt feelings, that's what I want.

Counselor: How do you think when you think of aborting, how do you feel?

Client: *(Pause.)* There would be a relief. I would feel relieved that the problem is over and — it's just that little idea that that might have been a baby, that could have been a baby, that maybe I wouldn't have the right to take the life away.

Counselor: When you think of that, do any other thoughts come to your mind?

Client: Well, like it's not right to take a life away. *(Pause.)* You know though, I wonder if I'm so much worried about the baby and taking its life away, as to how I feel about taking his life away; I'm more worried about me and how I'm going to handle it because what chance — I mean the kid — the world doesn't need any more kids, and it isn't a baby yet; it's just like if I would have used the pill, the egg is fertilized but it doesn't implant — that's just like it could have been a life.

Counselor: I had a feeling a moment ago when you mentioned the fertilized egg, that in a sense life isn't created; life simply ends.

Client: Life isn't created — say that again.

Counselor: Life isn't created; it simply ends.

Client: Ends? I guess I don't know what you mean — life isn't created, but I guess I don't understand why it doesn't begin.

Counselor: Well, look, you sensed a feeling that almost with all living things, there isn't any real start; there's only a stop. The egg is fertilized.

Client: In a way, except I can almost see the point of conception, as a starting.

Counselor: And yet you're saying to yourself that even if it had happened several times but you did not know it . . .

Client: Yeah, in that case it would be fine. I wouldn't think twice about it.

Counselor: So it isn't so much the fact of what happened it's your knowing about it.

Client: Yeah, sure, absolutely, if I didn't know, I . . .

Counselor: And somehow you managed to upset yourself.

Client: Or if I were to have a miscarriage or something and not find out until afterwards, that would have given me no qualms.

Counselor: We've kind of run into a spot here because we have run out of time. We could reschedule you for later today or early tomorrow because it sounds like to me that you are kind of in the middle of working this out.

Client: I'd like to come back.

Counselor: Maybe one of the things that you might give a little thought to is how you manage to upset yourself in a situation such as knowing about this.

Client: OK.

Following the counseling session, Dr. Carlson asked the client to share some of her feelings concerning this counseling session. Her reaction to the session provides valuable insights into the counseling process from the vantage point of the client.

Counselor: Well, Pat, I want to thank you very much for working with us. I'd like to get some of your reactions in terms of what happened.

Client: The feeling I had at the end was that I was really thinking clearly about this and a lot of the upset was gone. I had a couple of roads in which to think clearly, in which I hadn't before, particularly about the thing about the anger and how I was mad that this had to happen to me and I was letting that keep me from sitting down and making my decision, and the part about life ending naturally with my never knowing about it is fine, but with my decision, for some reason, I think it's not right. I really want to think about that a lot more.

Counselor: Do you have any idea of what would happen if you walked out of here? What your feelings would have been, your thinking would have been?

Client: Well, with the feeling that, "OK, I'm on my way now; I've got something to hold onto, something to work on, whereas I had myself not having anything before. I was just coming to two dead ends with both of them just not good alternatives." I felt that, "All right now; I can sit down and think about it," and I would have sat down and thought about it before coming back.

Counselor: What about other parts of the session? What other reactions do you have?

Client: Throughout the whole session, I didn't feel coerced one way or the other that you were moralizing or trying to get me to go one way or the other. Once I got mad when you were talking about the anger because I didn't want to let it go; you were pointing out to me how it really wasn't helping me.

Counselor: How did you get angry?

Client: Because I felt, "I want to keep this anger, and I can't let go of it." You were telling me something I didn't want to hear, mainly that I had to take the responsibility and make the decision, and I was mad.

Counselor: So the anger was the thing you needed to keep, knowing you were pregnant. And when you saw that, suddenly there was going to be a change in you then you began to get pissed at me.

Client: I was a little mad for that reason.

Counselor: How did you get mad?

Client: Because I said, "Watch out; you're going to have to make a decision." I said to myself, "Watch him; he's going to make you sit down and make that decision." I didn't want to.

Counselor: What else about that session?

Client: I felt relaxed with you. At first, I didn't know that, being as it was in a real pregnancy. I was sort of afraid that perhaps I was playing a game and so forth, but it didn't come to that. I got down to some real feelings and felt as if it were a real session. I don't know if you contributed to that; anyway, it didn't turn out to be a game I was playing. I thought of you as a counselor, not someone sitting there role-playing. One thing I completely forgot — this is being video-taped.

Counselor: There seemed to be a little hesitancy in the beginning. How did you feel in the opening moments of the session?

Client: That it was role-play — I was trying to psyche out what somebody seeing a counselor for the first time would be doing.

Counselor: That's a very interesting experience for myself because I kept debating whether I ought to go through with the structuring or resource start, and the funny thing was after I got in here, I felt I couldn't possibly do anything else but do it. I guess because it's generally the kind of structuring I do to my own clients; it's the type of structuring I do in the practicum that particularly we're being viewed on tape; I couldn't bring myself just to start, starting my setting structure when I came in.

Client: Yeah, I was knocked off a little bit . . .

Counselor: You weren't expecting that.

Client: No, I wasn't. I did know ahead of time though. I wonder what would have happened if I would have said, "No I'd rather not be on that tape."

Counselor: What do you think would have happened?

Client: Perhaps you would have said — I don't know, what would you have said? What would you have done?

Counselor: I would have tried to move it into counseling-wise, therapy-wise, and your feelings about it, how you generated your feelings. What else about the session?

Client: A general feeling that I was being helped.

Counselor: You mentioned that you were angry during the therapy when you saw a change, facing the pregnancy. Were there any points in the session when you felt uncomfortable or things were not running smoothly, or you were getting negative feelings?

Client: No, I think that was the only point when that happen.

Counselor: Now to understand you accurately, that was more your response in realizing that you're limited to really move anywhere for your own therapeutic lead. You need to give up the anger so you can begin to work up to the things which are facing you. It didn't really have to do with anything which I was doing realistically, in a reality.

Client: No. You mean . . .

Counselor: Look, you played this role a couple times before and one of them you got three-fifths off.

Client: Oh, and that was because of his right . . .

Counselor: The role he chose for pleasure.

Client: Yes, I understand. No, it was because of the content when I realized I had to do but because of the way you were directing questions at me, the attitude I felt you had or anything like that.

Counselor: What were your feelings towards me as a human being during the session?

Client: I was pretty wrapped up in myself, but I felt that this is someone who cares and wants to help me. And once you got going, I also got a respect for you. Some of the things you brought out I thought, "Yes, this is what I need." I got a respect for your ability to help me too and felt very comfortable with you.

Counselor: You're just finishing up a Master's now, hopefully moving out soon to the world of work, possibly a position where you may be facing these things on a daily basis, a weekly basis possibly. Whether there were things done here or not done would be helpful possibly.

Client: Now the only difference was that it was a short session. Ideally, I think it should have been a little longer as you found out I was just getting into something where it had an end.

Counselor: How did you feel at that moment? Here you are facing an almost crucial point and . . .

Client: Yeah, I wanted to continue, but, of course, I realized that we had to end it. In a real situation, I would have felt sort of frustrated if I would have had to stop at that point.

Counselor: That probably must have happened.

Client: I was going to say that must have happened. But the one thing you did say was "later today or tomorrow" which made me feel that we could get right back into it.

Counselor: Now why do you think I put it that way?

Client: You felt I was on to something that you really wanted to help me with.

Counselor: There is a time pressure when you find out — what does that mean when there is a time pressure?

Client: To have had to wait a week or three or four days would have been bad.

Counselor: If you were to go ahead and decide on abortion, it would have been very important to move rapidly — you would have already been eight weeks along, maybe ten, so that puts it into a very urgent category. If you would have decided to bear the child and then solve the problems of keep, place, and marriage, then it would not have been so urgent. I have kind of one last question. Do you have any questions to ask before we spring this one?

Client: No.

Counselor: Pat — she comes back maybe once, twice, three times, whatever it takes to help her work it through. What's your best guess now, considering that time has gone by, the decision is made. What was that decision?

Client: To have an abortion. I'd be almost positive after having been in.

Counselor: How do you know that?

Client: (*Pause.*) I just have the feeling that I would have one. True, I'd have the feeling of killing a life — just in that little bit, the last part we talked about. I have a feeling that I'd have the abortion.

Counselor: Does that really make a difference?

Client: Sort of, maybe, that I'm doing what I wanted to do and that just helped me to say, "Yeah, that's right."

Counselor: What do you think — both as a human being and as a gal in this type of situation, as a human being and also in terms of a professional counselor? Do you think it fair to move in and give a little push now and then, and is that what happened when I brought this up?

Client: You might have given a little push, but I think it came from me because I think what you said I was saying. I don't think you put anything in from outside; I think it was just from you.

Counselor: You mean I sort of put in the words which were so close to the surface?

Client: Yeah, that's what I felt. You didn't say anything about how you felt. You stated what I had just said. And I definitely feel that that is the way to go and one shouldn't push in a certain direction.

Counselor: Yet I bet if we look back, there would be a lot of people watching the segment and feel that I had pushed even so gently.

Client: I guess there's a line there and I don't know if we crossed it or not by simply trying to tell me what I said and help me really clarify my thoughts and add a tinge of your own into it. I don't feel you really crossed it but just a shade; I'm not sure.

Counselor: And yet you don't sense any big reaction to it, a big negative reaction to it.

Client: No, not at all, no. Yes if you did push, if that's what you're saying. If you did push, no I didn't get any big reaction. *(Laugh.)*

Counselor: Because I sense that not only were you heading in that direction but I sense myself that that was a little added ingredient and that it was not really a very conscious thing on my part, that it is a philosophical notion and it just seemed to me that sharing this with you, giving you a chance to think about it might result in your being able to use this to accept doing apparently what you haven't. Almost doing it but not quite. It was as if I was giving you just maybe a little support here. Now how do you respond to this?

Client: I can see that maybe that is what you were doing. I can say that at the time it was definitely a positive thing — facilitating.

Counselor: And only you can tell me and you said it was where you were headed and what I said was already a part of you. Does it still seem that way?

Client: Yes.

Counselor: And yet it's funny when I come back and say that I sense where you were moving, but I wasn't sensing that the precise concept was quite a part of you. I sense the concept that maybe you had never quite thought of that baby.

Client: I guess I felt that it had come out of me because if I hadn't quite thought of it, still when you said it, it seemed to me as if it were part of me, as if it was natural, even though in those exact terms I never really thought of it. It would fit into what I was thinking and feeling.

Counselor: And I had no notion in my own ideas and thinking. If you were going to reject it, I had the notion, in that sense, that it would be a part that fit. This fits in the notion that I have so strong, from the psychological point of view, the anger point of view, the function of point of view that people feel and what they do is a function of their beliefs, of their philosophies and the way they look around themselves and how they think about them.

Client: I was just thinking it over, relating it to what I have done in the session, and I can see that I was going to, eventually; my action would cover up my points of view of the world and my beliefs.

Counselor: I bet that surprised you when I asked you that. What do you think I would have done if you headed in the direction of bearing the child?

Client: I feel that you would have been perfectly accepting of that.

alex: freedom and identity through grass

or: are you kidding me?

Alex, a seventeen-year-old high-school senior, was referred to me by a former client. His presenting concern was that life was generally meaningless, few people understood him and his friends, and that dope and "funky blues music" were not only the best outlets for his feelings but were also the vehicles through which he would become a free person. Moreover, he indicated that after he was arrested for smoking marijuana, he subsequently developed "paranoid" or suspicious feelings over being caught again.

Alex blamed society's hypocrisy for his feelings of depression and alienation, but, for the most part, he blamed his parents for their inability to empathize with him. He identified strongly with a group of "long-haired-bearded-cool-with-it" guys who were searching for personal meaning and an authentic existential existence. He believed that the "pill or drug culture" offered him a set of meaningful personal relationships with persons who were also suffering from feelings of alienation, loneliness, and misunderstanding. For Alex, straight persons were living in their heads and were not tuned into the human condition.

A number of Alex's specific problems were identified over twelve counseling sessions spread over an eight-month period. Among these concerns were:

1. Excessive use of marijuana as a means of psychological escape
2. Feelings of worthlessness, depression, and internalized hostility
3. Poor academic performance
4. Influence of peer-group pressure to conform
5. Relationships with members of the opposite sex
6. Relationships with parents and other family members

On the issue of marijuana, Alex was able to articulate much empirical evidence in support of his views. His knowledge of the subject was thorough. Initially, our talks about using marijuana centered on a means of getting "high" or "kicks." Since at one level, given the status of present empirical evidence, moderate smoking may have few psychologically or physiologically harmful effects, I could not logically argue against this point. I could only point out the legal implications involved in getting caught. Alex agreed with me in words but I really believed that the chances of being busted a second time were so low that they could be disregarded.

Essentially, I supported Alex's idea that the moderate use of marijuana was not an inherently evil or pernicious behavior. But I did confront him with his stupid belief that the heavy smoking of "grass" as a means of "escaping conformity, academic pressures and parental control into a free and authentic existence was pure and simple 'bullshit.' " In relatively simple language, I directly and forcefully pointed out to him that "smoking pot" was probably one of the most ineffective means for him to counter feelings of loneliness, alienation, worthlessness, and the like. I informed him that while he was "sky high" on pot or any other "goddamned drug or symbol," he would be in a relatively poor position to counteract, contradict, or deal effectively with his feelings. In one sense, he was doing an excellent job of avoiding constructive action which would have a more long-lasting and positive effect on his development.

For several years, Alex had blamed his parents for the negative feelings he held about himself. He told me that they were too restrictive of his freedom. Moreover, he could not stand their yelling and screaming at him when he acted in defiance of them. There was evidence that Alex's father indiscriminately criticized him and, at the same time, indoctrinated him with the belief that he was a worthless and incompetent kid. Even though Alex's home environment was not at all to his liking, he did not have to become inordinately depressed or emotionally upset. I pointed out several facts to Alex:

1. That his father acted stupidly by putting him down was an indication that the father was personally disturbed; his put-downs were just a manifestation of his nutty thinking and emotions.
2. He was making a mistake in believing blindly those things his father said without really evaluating them for himself.
3. There was no evidence that he was worthless.
4. His father did have a right to be obnoxious or neurotic.

At first, Alex had a hard time accepting his father's self-defeating tendencies, but, in time, he gained a greater acceptance of the father, was able to discriminate between the father's sound and unsound judgments, and was able to assert himself more calmly and effectively.

As a result of Alex's hard work on and practicing of many of the homework assignments I gave him (among the most significant of which was, of course, mastering the ABC technique), many positive changes were evidenced in his present functioning. First, he reduced significantly his smoking of marijuana from about seven times a week to about once a month. Second, Alex began to cultivate new friends, thus modifying his dependence on his peer group. Third, he initiated healthy hetero-sexual activities. Fourth, he improved in his academic performance. Fifth, and most important, he admitted to a feeling of well-being and a greater control over his own life. Alex now seems sufficiently committed to a rational-realistic philosophy or personal orientation towards life. And I believe he has captured for himself a fundamental grasp of the process of living at a very early age. Incidentally, several follow-up sessions eight months later revealed that the above gains were sustained by Alex.

dianne: towards self-realization through re counseling

Dianne C. was twenty-four years old, employed as a school teacher, and had been divorced from her husband recently. Prior to her RE coun-seling experience, Dianne had undergone an existential-analytical coun-seling experience which provided her with some understandings to her "here-and-now functioning." The focus of her previous counseling had been primarily on the expression of key emotions, some of which she had repressed. Although she had made some significant personal gains, she continued to suffer from frequent depression. Moreover, she ex-pressed a great concern over her own ability to relate intimately with men, and, specifically, she was not able to experience an orgasm during coitus. Dianne also complained of excessive guilt over her sexual activity.

Her compulsive strivings for perfection in herself and others were given much attention in RE counseling. Unresolved parental conflicts were explored as well. In the course of about fifteen counseling sessions over a six-month period, Dianne was thoroughly trained in the use of ABC analysis as it applied to her sexual activity, her interaction with her parents, her divorce, and her feelings of guilt and depression. She also was taught to focus on sexually arousing stimuli during coitus which would enhance the probability of her experiencing an orgasm — which she finally was able to achieve.

The following is a verbatim interchange between Dianne and me. This was a special session which occurred four months after the coun-seling sessions had terminated. The session was recorded specifically for this book with the purpose of capturing the evaluation and description of the counseling process from the client's point of view. As Dianne related her perceptions of her own personal growth to me during this session, I gave thought to both the specific RE interventions and her achieving a higher level of personal functioning. My thoughts were mainly on her progress in terms of the various dimensions of self-realization: Inner directedness, existentiality, feeling reactivity, spontaneity, self-regard, self-acceptance, nature of man, synergy, acceptance of aggression, and capacity for intimate contact. I believe her words are expressions of tremendous growth.

Counselor: Dianne, now you have had an opportunity to experience what is typically called rational-emotive counseling. You came in about a year or so ago and had in the neighborhood of fifteen sessions spread out over an eight-month period. In this session, I would appreciate your reactions regarding: (a.) some of the things you have learned about yourself as a result of that experience and (b.) the ways you overcame some of the personal concerns you presented during our first few counseling sessions.

Client: I think, first of all, the thing which has been particularly exciting to me was that through this particular phase of my life, I have begun to assume greater control of some of my own change and my own progress. I have been through some therapy before and it was tremendously helpful and brought me a long way and maybe prepared me for this. But in this process of applying some of the REC methods, I think the significance I see for myself is that I am more capable of assessing myself and situations more realistically and when I become upset, I am better able to move myself through it, being more in control of the processes within me. *(Inner Direction and Self-Acceptance)*

Counselor: In other words, as you experienced other forms of therapy, you discovered many things about yourself. You were able to understand more clearly some of the things that were sources of disturbance and some of the reasons or causes why you were disturbed. And you say that as a result of the RE experience, you were better able to learn some of the kinds of things you could do to get yourself functioning more effectively. In other words, you were better able to put into practice many of the ideas you learned about yourself as a result of previous counseling sessions. Is that about it?

Client: Yes, that's very accurate. And I'm just suddenly finding that a lot of it had to do with me and that no counselor was doing anything magic to me. It had a lot to do with how I perceived things and what I could put together for myself.

Counselor: So that through this type of process you were able to get in touch with the fact — the most important fact — that therapists are not magicians or super-human persons.

Client: I've been fairly aware that it had a lot to do with the counselee, but I just found the REC more practical and something that I could get a handle on. I could get a handle on some of these techniques and use them within myself when I'd be willing. Sometimes, I'd find myself resisting because it was easier to avoid applying some of these things to myself.

Counselor: Yes, there is this normal tendency to experience difficulty when you're in the process of growing or simply to resist that process.

Client: Right.

Counselor: By now, of course, you are aware of the REC interpretation of the law of inertia. But in spite of the tendency to resist, you were able to persist in your efforts or get back into the "growth groove."

Client: Yeah, like I know that sometimes if I really work myself into a depression, I realize that I have literally talked myself into it, and I realize that I have the capacity and skill to bring myself out of it. But I discover that maybe I do enjoy that depression a bit right then or get some attention from others. And so I almost refuse to bring myself out of it even though I know I could.

Counselor: That's interesting. How do you finally overcome your depression?

Client: Well, first of all, one thing I'd say I have learned is to acknowledge that if I am depressed, it's OK to be there, and *so what if* I am depressed sometimes, so long as I don't allow myself to stay there for an unhealthy period of time. Then, once I realize I've been there long enough and that I don't really like being there, I begin to assess how I got depressed in the first place, what kind of demands I was putting on other people that were maybe unfair, what kinds of demands I was putting on myself, checking out some irrelevant kinds of data that really aren't what I make them to be, and I suppose then, I wouldn't say I take myself into a happy state or into a real euphoria, but at least I get myself out of the depression into sort of just a normal, relatively calm state. And then I'm more ready to receive other kinds of experiences which might help me feel happier. *(Acceptance of Aggression)*

Counselor: So you say you still have the tendency to get yourself feeling upset at times but are capable of dealing effectively with your negative feelings.

Client: And I know I can and that's significant. You know, my sister, for instance, when she does not have things going the way she would like them to go becomes severely depressed. She then has to have other people to bring her out. When I get depressed, sometimes its nice to have a friend to talk to, and its even nice to cry on somebody's shoulder once in a while, but I know that I don't have to do that and I know that sometimes I don't even choose to do that. Most importantly, I can live through it and come out of it feeling pretty healthy and that's a good place to be. *(Inner Direction and Self-Acceptance)*

Counselor: Can you give some specific examples of problems or personally self-defeating situations you confronted and worked through?

Client: Oh, I'd say several, and I wouldn't say they were all worked through completely, yet I feel very confident that I am in the process — but I think this is significant in itself that I know for sure now that it's not a matter of complete solutions or a total getting it together. There are things that I will probably be working on — some of these same things probably I'll be working on for a long time and perhaps some new things as I mature and change. I suppose originally I was overly concerned with perfection. I definitely demanded perfection in myself and perfection in others and all the implications that follow. Also, I am still working through dependence on my parents and the related implications. A third area is my own comfort and natural feelings related to sex and sexual behavior and sorting what's appropriate for me and comfortable for me and what it is I've been telling myself about that. Those would be the three main areas with some subareas. I think they're somewhat related because like, for instance, my parents had a tremendous influence on me; it's like they expected me to be a perfect child and so I began to expect that of myself and, then obviously placed those kinds of demands in operation. They were impossible for me to maintain. And, then, all the guilt and self-blaming that go with not being able to be perfect so I put that on other people expecting those same things in them. That gave me a double problem. I have some talents and some skills and I can do things quite well, and because of that, I would make heavy demands on other people who may have had fewer skills or talents to work with — I was very hard on them and quite judgmental. *(Self-Acceptance, Time Competence)*

Counselor: How were you able to overcome these difficulties?

Client: Well, on the matter of my parents, which I believe I am working through rather successfully, although I can still disturb myself over them, the REC has been tremendously helpful. The ABC analysis applied to my parents was certainly beneficial. I finally realized that I have the right to choose for myself what my behavior is, and if anyone else chooses to react to that, it is their reaction. Now if it's a neurotic reaction — and this is tremendously applicable to my parents since they do tend to disturb themselves considerably over their children's behavior, I now realize it is their problem and that I don't have to give them additional information to upset themselves over, but if they should come across this information or through conversation things come up, I am in a place where I can accept their disturbing themselves — and that's OK. Now, this frees me to choose behaviors that are very different from what they would expect in their value system, which, by the way, is less than perfect. I'm much more able to say, "Damn, I wish I wouldn't have done that or I wish I wouldn't have said that or I wish I wouldn't have behaved that way, but that's OK, the next time around I'll try to improve myself. I don't suffer as much over things which I have done to my parents. *(Existentiality, Spontaneity, Self-Regard)*

Counselor: In other words, if you make a mistake with your parents or if you do behave in such a way that they disturb themselves, you simply say to yourself, "Look, I made a mistake and next time I'll try to improve it, but I don't have to beat myself over the head needlessly because I did make a mistake or because they became disturbed."

Client: Right. I feel pretty comfortable with the whole parent thing and the way I reconstructed that personally. I have also improved in my relationship with other people, where if I did something that really was crappy or felt badly about, I just would suffer with it, magnify it, dwell on it, and remember it. I still have a tendency to do that occasionally with men, but, generally speaking, with relationships, say in my work, I'm much more able to say, "Chalk that one up for a bad show," and we'll see where it goes from here. It makes me much less self-conscious and much less compulsive about monitoring myself. Therefore I'm more spontaneous and probably much more easy to be with. *(Spontaneity, Self-Acceptance)*

Counselor: You're reacting much more spontaneously at work and more spontaneously with members of the opposite sex, but you say there is room for improvement in the latter category.

Client: I would say that the spontaneity in me is one of the major changes that I and other people could notice. I have often been known as a very serious type, rather tight, and very uncomfortable if anyone would touch me — physically. I was especially self-conscious about my body, and now I feel very comfortable about my body most of the time. *(Self-Acceptance)*

Counselor: Many men and women have berated themselves for not being perfect or thoroughly competent physically. Could you indicate the process that you go through in order to feel better about your own body, your own physical being?

Client: That's been a long process and one which I am still working on. But I'm comfortable with it because it's coming and I don't see any need to rush it. I know first I was beginning to, well, for me I wasn't even aware that I was attractive; I wasn't aware that men noticed me, so first I began noticing that men noticed me and that made me feel good; it was reinforcing and then —

Counselor: You mean, it was nice that men noticed you.

Client: Yes, it was very nice — I used to put down my body partially because of some things that a man told me at one time; he was getting on me for having small breasts, and I realize that a lot of that had to do with his ego and what he was into. I began accepting my breasts and realizing that they were what I had and I was not going to change or alter that fact. Also, I took it upon myself to get more information about sex. I discovered that size doesn't make any difference in being able to be excited or whatever and, then, as I've been feeling better about that, I've been less tense with men concerning my breasts and, therefore, have found out that many men like them because they're firm, because they're smooth, and so all of a sudden the size is not so significant. Initially, I had to work through things like being able to tell myself that they are not so bad, and even if they were, that didn't have anything to do with me enjoying myself sexually. That thinking freed me up enough to experiment a little bit and test out whether they were OK. *(Self-Acceptance, Capacity for Intimacy)*

Counselor: So, in other words, you stopped telling yourself that you were horrible because you had small breasts and decided to test this hypothesis out; you soon found that it was not so bad having small breasts. As a matter of fact, it was *irrelevant.*

Client: And it would still be nice to have larger breasts but it's not terrible; it's not catastrophic; it's OK the way it is. The other thing I learned to do is learn to choose clothing that maybe brings out my best features. I noticed that when I felt more comfortable about my body, I became increasingly feminine; I mean increasingly warm. *(Capacity for Intimacy)*

Counselor: You seem to be saying that "since I have been able to deindoctrinate myself, that is, deindoctrinating much of the bullshit I've been telling myself for years about myself, condemning myself, putting myself down, I feel much more positively about myself. As a result I am becoming more spontaneous and more capable of relating to people, both men and women."

Client: I'm beginning to think that how I feel about myself sexually has been very closely related to many other things in my life. Because now that I'm more comfortable with myself sexually, I'm more comfortable in many, many other areas. The other thing is — the most fantastic thing is — that suddenly it hit me not too long ago that I am in control of it, that I used to be so up-tight because I thought men were up to games, up to all kinds of things. And all of a sudden, I realized that I am intelligent enough to sort through what the games are and see them for what they are. And I can choose anything I want to sexually; I can react at many levels with men; I can sort that for myself; I don't have to be afraid of games — you know, games that are played on you sometimes. *(Capacity for Intimacy)*

Counselor: That's not your problem if someone else plays a game.

Client: Right, and I have the capacity to sort that out. I can better understand and accept others. I can begin determining where I'm coming from in response. Maybe sometimes I'm in the mood for games. *(Nature of Man)*

Counselor: Yes, it sounds like this has a lot to do with your ability to appraise situations more accurately. Your reactions to many social situations are more spontaneous.

Client: Exactly. And I guess why it was such a fantastic revelation in the sexual area, because I used to feel so hung-up in that particular one. In that area, I was so up-tight that it was a real beautiful feeling to find that I could choose, I could select, and I could monitor and it wasn't a somebody doing-me-in-kind of thing all the time. *(Capacity for Intimacy)*

Counselor: Yeah, I think this sexual thing was symbolic of your self-defined lack of womanness at one time. I think you have turned that around a great deal. In other words, you changed many of the meanings you ascribed to feminine symbols. For instance, you've been attacking your perfectionistic beliefs which you imposed upon yourself and others, and you also are attacking rather successfully this notion of your lack of sexuality and your inability to relate to others more intimately.

Client: Well, I think as I increasingly became comfortable with myself, I could increasingly touch people in a very personal, genuine way, and people could receive it very comfortably from me. But the thing that was still hanging me up was when I would touch people in a sexual way and to me there is still a distinction. I don't know whether there should or shouldn't be, but for me, there still is. I can touch and extend myself freely and comfortably in nonsexual ways, be comfortable with touching or being touched, and it's only when there are sexual implications that I still have to practice my ABCs. But that's OK because I think that one of the most exciting things for me to realize is the fact that I recognize that I am in process because that speaks for the whole perfectionistic thing. Before I was struggling to get there, to get to some perfect state and it's very important for me to realize that I'm not going to get there, I'm going to work different things through and then I'm going to begin to pick up different things and work them through. And I have improved much in the whole sexual arena.

Counselor: In other words, now you're coming into closer contact with the process of living, and you're not necessarily focusing all your energies on achieving perfectionistic goals. "I must be something great or I must achieve a total state of sanity by this afternoon." In other words, you're saying, "It's more important for me to focus greater attention on living and the process of life rather than on long-term goals." I see that as one of your major gains. That is being able to rid yourself of needless, self-defeating neurotic tunnel vision.

Client: There's such a difference in my experience particularly. I used to concentrate tremendously on the past and on the future. I would spend many hours making scrapbooks, reminiscing, trying to keep in touch with old friends. I would also look forward to the time when I would be a mother and all the things that I thought were so important in my future. And now, suddenly, I have a keenly increased capacity to be where I am right now and enjoy what is right now. Occasionally feeling a sentiment for the past but not needing to cling to old friends or old situations. I have much more capacity to get into new situations and to make new friends. I almost prefer this because there are so many interesting things happening right now. *(Time Competence)*

Counselor: Very good. I am also interested in your reaction to rational-emotive counseling?

Client: I find that it's very, very helpful, for this reason: because you can begin to think for yourself. Now I am able to take charge of myself. I think, though, that it takes a very skillful counselor to use it—it's deceptive on the surface, it looks like you apply a series of steps one, two, and three. I know that in trying to use it and using it, it is very easy to learn the basics, but I think the skill comes when a counselor can help the counselee take it to the deeper things — the basic irrational ideas or beliefs. If it doesn't get to that level, then it's just a technique that steers a person away from the basic things. What I really like about it is that I can apply the concepts in a situation where I'm depressed and don't want to be or angry at someone when there is no call for my being angry. I find that I can say, "Now wait a minute; what is this that I'm telling myself about this situation; what kinds of demands am I putting on them; what kinds of demands am I putting on myself?" Now I can really process it and deal with many situations where I would have previously been disturbed. *(Feeling Reactivity)*

Counselor: In other words, you've become proficient in the use of ABC technique. What I'm also interested in, Dianne, is your reaction to the active, directive approach as opposed to a more passive, nondirective one.

Client: I remember thinking had I initially come into counseling, that you probably would have offended me a lot and I would have been offended by the forcefulness, by the strong language and that sort of thing. Now I was at a place where it didn't bother me as much. Your comment was that I would have worked that through, and I can see that now that you could use that content and apply the concepts of REC to it. I think the thing that I finally realized was that, again, the responsibility that I needed to take. For instance, at first I would sometimes sit and let you say, "Now, does this sound right; does this seem to apply?" Where sometimes it wouldn't and I was sort of looking at a counselor as sort of a person who was a know-it-all. I finally had to realize that you were saying some things that were close and it was up to me to clarify and to restate. It took me a couple of times to realize my responsibility in the relationship. I think that if a counselor is on the right track, this is a really fast method of getting to some places if the person is ready to handle it. I think I would be frightened a little bit in terms of counselors who didn't know what they were doing using this method. You can get to some basic things very quickly. In my experiences as a school counselor, sometimes people aren't ready for it.

Counselor: Yes, there are times when we must be extremely sensitive to that. You usually encounter one or two people who have a tendency to become upset with this approach. Therefore, we must vary our delivery. That is, sometimes we must be very warm and understanding and take the time to teach about the counseling. We are not indiscrimately active, directive, and forceful.

Client: I thought it was interesting too that you did digress for a couple of weeks to get into some historical things that were important for me to learn about. You brought in some other techniques and some other ways of operating.

Counselor: Yes, I thought it might be appropriate for you to gain some insights into the antecedents of your present behavior. So we took a more Freudian-type analytical-interpretive approach for a while to help you uncover the origins of some of your believing, present-day believing and thinking. We would call that insight number one in REC; that's the usual type of Freudian insight — how the past influences the present. A second type of insight was for you to discover how you sustained those early negative experiences which now occur in the form of your beliefs or what you're telling yourself. The idea is to become aware of irrational sentences or thoughts you use as well as more rational ways of believing, thinking about yourself. But, most importantly, it is the third type of insight I think you've gained. That is when you concluded, "I'm in the process of growing." Or, more specifically, the fact that in order to get better, in order to develop yourself, you've got to work; you've got to practice, work and practice, and work and practice *ad infinitum*. Usually, a lot of therapies and counseling approaches focus on insight number one, and sometimes they get to insight number two but they often deemphasize insight number three, which is really the most important. The third type of insight is the one which enables a therapeutic process which can be a highly intellectual and emotive one to become a very pragmatic action-oriented one.

Client: Well, I think on my part that was one of the most important things that I got out of this for this reason. As I look around and as I look at myself, I know that for as long as I've been in some kind of therapy, there are still some of the original things there; they didn't go magically away. But the difference is I can accept myself and accept that there are still some problematic areas. And I can accept the fact that I am working and don't need immediate solutions. Furthermore, I realize that maybe some of my problems may never be worked out. But the difference is self-acceptance and the constructive action. *(Self-Regard, Self-Affirmation)*

Counselor: It seems to me that you're cognizant of a normal tendency to disturb yourself, and you seem willing to accept that. That's a major step. And it's really important that you do understand that we have not arrived at a state of absolute euphoria or self-actualization. After all, we are not living in heaven. The fact of the matter is, that you are in the process of becoming a more reasonable person; you are working very hard, judging from the personal gains you have made. It is interesting that you do evaluate the fact that you are working rather hard in very positive terms in spite of some of the difficulties you still encounter in the process. It's not all pleasure, is it?

Client: Something I noticed just recently. I used to have the fear that I would become very analytical, that I would start dissecting everything that happened; that was a real concern and just this weekend I went into a depression and then last night I was feeling very good and I realized that in both instances I responded very well and came through it, reacting to whatever were my feelings and accepting the fact that I was uncomfortable, but it was not horrible for me to feel this way. My negative feelings have not stopped me from reacting reasonably, and it just makes me know a little bit more what my reaction is all about. *(Acceptance of Aggression)*

Counselor: Well, it's been nice that we had this opportunity to sit down once again. I really appreciated your reactions to the RE counseling process. Very rarely do we have the opportunity to sit down with our clients in this way, although it probably is a good idea to take this opportunity more often because it gives me great insight into my own way of operating. Most importantly, it helps me capture more of what you are all about at a later point. Are there any final concluding remarks?

Client: I was thinking about one thing related to the counselor's style. There is, as I perceive it, in this style of therapy, less of that enveloping warmth, less of unconditional positive regard. I'm not sure that's bad; it's basically there, if the person basically realizes that you are concerned for them and working with them. I think if there's too much of the other, there will be a more of a dependence on the therapist. You literally force the person into thinking for himself. *(Inner Direction)*

Counselor: Let me react to that. I would say that we're not overly warm and overly expressive and emotive like some of our contemporary humanistically-oriented counselors and therapists. But on the matter of unconditional positive regard, I might disagree a little bit. Because I think we would probably offer more than most counselors. I think we accept the person's right to his own disturbances; we do not evaluate his worth in negative terms because he is neurotic, stupid, or psychotic. We accept that he is alive and that we can deal with this person in spite of his self-defeating tendencies, in spite of what he does and says. But when we intervene, we intervene in a serious, directive manner. Sometimes one might erroneously associate an RE counselor's directiveness and activity with unconditional negative regard. This is a mistake. We unconditionally accept that a person has the right to be what he is. But, also, if that person wants to change and is willing to change and wants that counselor to help him change, most RE counselors will, in fact, get off their ass and get involved with him. Although we are criticized by some, we accept the criticism and work like hell to help our clients grow. As a matter of fact, I think a little bit more than a lot of counselors and therapists.

six ✳ rational-emotive counseling in groups

To this point, the major emphasis of this book has been RE counseling on a one-to-one basis. The counselor-client dyad served as the prime interpersonal context for individual growth and development. However, the context for personal growth is not limited to the dyad. Personal development also can occur effectively in other meaningfully-structured situations, such as in groups, classrooms, business organizations, and religious organizations. In this chapter, the implications of rational emotive theory for group counseling and guidance are explored.

group counseling: a point of view

Unlike many of the popular, highly expressive-emotive group interactions (Lowen, 1969; Perls, 1969; Schultz, 1971) exemplified by encounter groups, gestalt groups, and the like, rational-emotive group counseling persistently emphasizes the balance between cognitive-didactic, experiential-emotive, and behavioral processes. Moreover, well-planned and extensive systematic extra-counseling assignments are included routinely.

Few counselors and therapists who identify themselves with the current expressive-emotive group therapies stress, as do RE counselors, the necessity of structured and planned experiences outside of the therapeutic modality. Many of these counselors and therapists are obsessively compulsive about "here-and-now" processes within the group itself that

144

they may often overlook the client's functioning in the outside world. Oftentimes, they erroneously assume that the self-learnings occurring within the group will be transferred automatically to ouside situations. Rarely in these "one shot" or highly expressive-emotive encounters are the six growth stages attended to: awareness, exploration, commitment, skill development, skill refinement, and change and redirection. Most often, these group experiences (although intense but of short duration) focus on awareness and exploration of self and others, although in some instances, persons participating in emotive-evocative groups may make verbal commitments to growth. But, often, they do not avail themselves of later opportunities to develop and refine the personal-interpersonal skills necessary for effective living. The development of skills, as we have already seen, takes work and practice over a rather extended time frame.

The initial structuring of a rational-emotive group experience is, in part, dependent upon time, location, or situational variables. If the group encounters are to be short — for example, three to five two-hour sessions with a group of secondary teachers in their own school — it would not be expected that the group members would pass through the six stages of growth. Under these conditions (like other short-term groups), it could only be expected that the group participants might gain in awareness and exploration of self and others. It would be too much to expect a commitment for growth in only a relatively short period of time. Given, however, ten sessions over a four-month period, a more preferred mode for RE counselors, it would be reasonable to attend to all six growth stages relative to a specific set of individual or group concerns. In rational-emotive group counseling, the counselor emphasizes the importance of the client's *long-term* and *ongoing involvement and commitment* to the counseling process (Wolfe, 1972).

initiating the group

Following a relatively didactic orientation wherein he explicates rational-emotive theory and practice and the structure of the group experiences, the counselor proceeds to initiate the group process. Usually, the counselor will ask someone to volunteer to share an emotionally upsetting concern. The counselor then takes the initiative and proceeds to deal directly with that specific concern. For instance, he may demonstrate to that client the ABC method of problem analysis and confrontation. Considerable time might be spent on teaching the ABCs of emotional disturbance to the client while he is expressing and experiencing strong emotions. While the counselor works one-to-one with a member of the group, the other members are encouraged to attend to that process. The notion is that the other members, while focusing on the growth of another person, will experience and learn about the growth process vicariously. Ultimately, the counselor will encounter each member of the group on a one-to-one basis.

After having experienced the ABC theory of emotional disturbance for themselves, members of the group are encouraged by the counselor to serve as counselors. Active-directive but reasonable confrontations by group members are reinforced. Thus, the group moves into more of a member-interaction process in which the counselor stimulates, guides, and maintains more reasonable modes of member interaction.

reinforcing and maintaining the group

Once the group members have initiated desirable therapeutic activity, the counselor reinforces and encourages the continuation of such activity. The counselor reinforces group members for appropriate cognitive-affective self-disclosures and also reinforces constructive helping by other group members. Each group member functions as a helper at times and as a helpee at other times. One of the RE counselor's major functions is to maintain the balance between helper-helpee activity on the part of each member.

As group members become more proficient in the self-application of RE principles, they also will become more effective in their teaching of these principles to one another. When there is evidence that the group is moving towards this end, the RE counselor becomes less active and directive and assumes a more supporting, reflective and consulting role. But when it is necessary to intervene forcefully, he does not hesitate.

"i"-ness in re group counseling

In a rational-emotive group process, "we"-ness is deemphasized and "i"-ness emphasized. The notion that a group identity is better than an individual identity is not reinforced by RE counselors. When peer persuasion exists in RE groups, it is of the type that encourages one to be himself. Persons who experience a rational encounter group or an ongoing therapy group learn eventually that they do not need absolute and total love and approval from others for their emotional growth, although love and approval can contribute desirably to one's growth to some extent. Healthy interactions with others are unquestionably a desirable human condition. But our moments of loneliness and isolation should not be discounted, for in those periods, meaningful growth is often privately realized.

In REC groups, as in individual REC, much emphasis is placed on behavior outside of the counseling situation. The group is construed mostly as a vehicle through which a person can establish ultimately a more reasonable set of attitudes and behavior outside of the group. If, in the REC group process, there are signs of a person's being pushed into growth inhibiting conformity, the RE counselor will attempt to combat the threat by insisting that the client initiate constructive independent actions outside of the group.

In general, expressive-emotive groups that deeemphasize cognitive reconstruction outside of counseling assignments are of limited value for the person. True, many people receive benefit from their participation in these groups in that they attend to their real feelings and emotions. This is help, but it may be superficial and incomplete. Just because a man knows and is in touch with his hostile feelings towards his wife does not mean that he will deal effectively with those feelings. Moreover, there is the danger that he may indiscriminately manifest excessive hostility and then incorrectly associate it with negative treatment from others. To know one is angry is one thing; to accept and to manage one's anger and aggression is yet another thing. I believe most expressive-emotive counselors would go along with these ideas. And I am also sure they too inform their clientele that the indiscriminate expression of hostility is not in their best interest. But I am not sure that these counselors would didactically demonstrate to the client how he creates and maintains his hostile feelings and behavior and, most importantly, how he can control those self-defeating states effectively.

group leadership in rec

In a rational-emotive counseling or therapy group, there is little doubt who the group leader is: It is the counselor or therapist. RE theory applied to groups sharply contrasts those group theories assuming the position that the counselor or leader is just another group member who is there for his own growth and development (Egan, 1970). It is not to be denied that a counselor can grow as a result of his leadership in a group or that at times group members do operate as counselors or therapists. Ellis (1969) believes that the counselor's activity in a group context is not unusually different from his behavior in a one-to-one encounter. The counselor or therapist directs, teaches, and confronts each member or sets of members within the group actively. Essentially, the rational-emotive position involves intensive one-to-one counseling within the group context. Although certain exercises may be used to stimulate or heighten emotional reactivity from group members, these serve only as vehicles and play only a small role in the process. Growth games, extensive role-playing, and the like are deemphasized.

In my own practice of rational-emotive counseling with groups, I spend considerable time, sometimes the first two or three sessions, introducing the group members to the theory and practice of rational-emotive counseling. The rationale for such an orientation is to provide the group members with a cognitive-emotive-behavioral framework from which to understand the counseling group process. During this orientation period the clients are made aware of the basic tenets of rational-emotive theory, within the framework of the person in the environment model. Moreover, I give outside reading assignments augmenting the material presented during the orientation.

The orientation period consists of the following steps:

1. Introduction of the group members to the person-environment model as discussed in Chapter One
2. Explanation of the stages of the counseling process or client growth stages: awareness, exploration, commitment, skill development, skill refinement, redirection or change
3. Introduction of the rudiments of rational-emotive theory, such as the ABC theory of emotional disturbance and problem analysis
4. Description and discussion of some of the most commonly-held irrational ideas and their rational alternatives
5. Providing the group member with a description of the counselor's or leader's role—teaching, confronting, persuading, encouraging, intervening

rational-emotive guidance in groups

The flexibility of the RE system permits meaningful extensions to a variety of situations. Because of REC's strong didactic orientation, many of its principles can be conveyed through many media — films, books, video tape, audio tape, and lectures. Therefore, a person can become aware of RE theory and practice quite easily. Moreover, because RE formulations are practical and simplistic, they are easily translated into language that junior and senior high school students can come to understand.

Recently, Ellis (1969), through the Institute for Rational Living in New York City, has begun an elementary school for normal children. The philosophical-psychological base for that school is rational-emotive theory. Presently, research on the efficacy of this venture is being conducted.

In the Counseling and Guidance Department at Ohio State University (Tosi and Liggit, 1973), group guidance courses have been arranged through independent study whereby RE principles and practices are being employed in some junior high schools in the Columbus area. Research on the effectiveness of such RE group guidance is currently underway. Preliminary research reports do indicate that junior high school students are benefiting from the experience.

The RE group guidance intervention strategy incorporates both didactic and experiential components. Initially, RE group guidance is heavily didactic, but as time goes on, the process becomes more experiential. The students who participated in junior high school project were defined as discipline problems by teachers and administrators. Whether or not these definitions were reasonable, the students involved expressed numerous self-defeating emotions, behaviors, and thoughts, among which were tardiness, frequent classroom disruptions, reticence, underachievement, and parental conflicts. There were three phases to this particular RE guidance program.

phase one: the re orientation

The orientation consisted of four one-hour meetings during which the counselor explicated the ABC theory of emotional disturbance. Written materials and lectures were the primary means of communicating this basic RE principle. Sessions were divided into two periods — forty minutes of content presentation and twenty minutes of group discussion of the content.

Specific reading assignments covering the ABC theory were given which were to be done outside of the group. In addition, students were given the task of attending to and identifying specific situations that were sources of disturbance to them (focusing and discrimination training). They were also asked to record these events as well as their feelings. Finally, the students were introduced to the ten irrational ideas by the counselor.

phase two: re group interaction

Phase Two of RE group guidance is process oriented. First, the students discussed the ABC theory among themselves, giving personal examples of how the theory fits. Group members were encouraged by the counselor to give helpful suggestions and criticisms to one another. At the initial stage of Phase Two, most of the discussions focused on situations outside of the group. Later on, however, conflicts between group members were analyzed through the ABC method. There was an inside-the-group and an outside-the-group focus in Phase Two. The Group Interaction phase occurred within four one-hour sessions.

phase three: outside application

In this final phase, the central focus was not so much on member interaction as on individual application of RE principles to outside situations. In Phase Three, the members took on helper roles to the extent that they reinforced in one another rational thinking and application. This phase occurs over about four one-hour sessions.

The major value in introducing RE ideas into the junior high school or elementary schools through group guidance is that it provides the students with an understandable framework in which to analyze and confront many of the problems facing them. RE group guidance activities can be introduced to all students because it is not essential that RE guidance and counseling occur only on a one-to-one or a small-group basis. The counselor can work with thirty or forty students at one time. Though, during this time, there are one-to-one confrontations.

seven ✳ conclusion

A few final words are needed to bring this volume to a close. Personal development was emphasized throughout this presentation. I was careful, however, not to lose sight of the reality that personal development occurs within a social framework — whether that framework be a counseling relationship, a classroom situation, or whatever. I deliberately channeled my energy into the person and attempted to place the person at the center of the environments in which he interacts, for it is the person himself who has to establish a unique and rational identity if he is to achieve a personally effective independence of thought, feeling, and action.

The thesis developed in the preceding chapters portrayed the person as one who does not discover himself easily, or, for that matter, act authentically without great personal effort. In fact, most counselors and therapists eventually discover that their most "normal" clients require a great deal of their energy. Personal growth is by no means an "instant turn on." To become an authentic person or a rationally choosing human being, one must commit himself to a process of self-scrutiny and action that requires the virtual elimination of self-defeating and self-deceiving tendencies. Ultimately, one needs to know himself, accept himself, and affirm himself in the world. The rewards of an authentic or rational existence will not be a "total joy or euphoria." The fact of one's existence is, at times, nauseating — even though one may strive for personal happiness.

Figure 4 summarizes the major topics of the book. As you will recall, we started with the self-processes and the development of the self in the socio-cultural system. Then, we moved to the growth stages of the counseling process and the goals of that process. But, as we all know, effective growing does not come easily. Therefore, imposed between the self and its processes are the conditions under which growth can be realized and the interventions that stimulate and push persons toward those ends that appear reasonable. These growth stages and conditions as well as the interventions were interpreted in a counseling and phychotherapeutic framework. It is not necessary that effective personal growing take place only in a counseling relationship. The processes, conditions, and interventions explicated here are currently being applied in education, business, religious institutions, and other social institutions.

As an "intervention" or overall counseling strategy, I have chosen a rational-emotive viewpoint. For me, personally, this counseling or therapeutic approach directly penetrates quickly into the core of the person's cognitive, affective, and behavioral system. Most importantly, a rational-emotive counseling experience enables a person to learn the art and science of reconstructing his philosophic belief system. RE counselors, for the most part, actively strive to persuade their clients virtually to stop deceiving themselves and to force themselves, if necessary, into constructive action. As you may have already noticed, RE counseling is extremely active, directive, and forceful in substance.

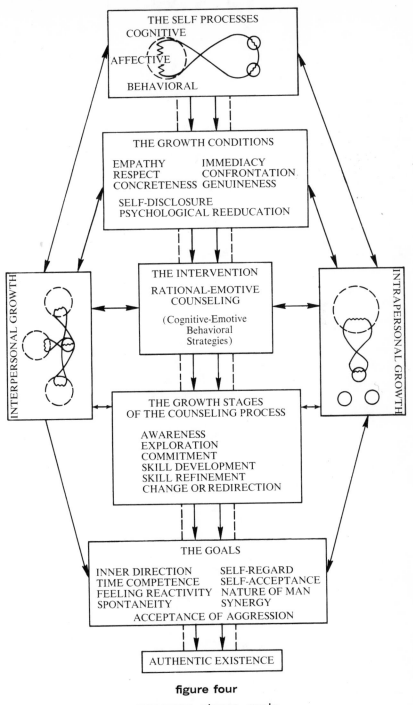

THE SELF PROCESSES
COGNITIVE
AFFECTIVE
BEHAVIORAL

THE GROWTH CONDITIONS

EMPATHY   IMMEDIACY
RESPECT   CONFRONTATION
CONCRETENESS   GENUINENESS

SELF-DISCLOSURE
PSYCHOLOGICAL REEDUCATION

INTERPERSONAL GROWTH

THE INTERVENTION

RATIONAL-EMOTIVE
COUNSELING

(Cognitive-Emotive
Behavioral
Strategies)

INTRAPERSONAL GROWTH

THE GROWTH STAGES
OF THE COUNSELING PROCESS

AWARENESS
EXPLORATION
COMMITMENT
SKILL DEVELOPMENT
SKILL REFINEMENT
CHANGE OR REDIRECTION

THE GOALS

INNER DIRECTION   SELF-REGARD
TIME COMPETENCE   SELF-ACCEPTANCE
FEELING REACTIVITY   NATURE OF MAN
SPONTANEITY   SYNERGY
ACCEPTANCE OF AGGRESSION

AUTHENTIC EXISTENCE

figure four

processes, stages, goals

153

references

Allen, T.W. "Effectiveness of Counselor Trainees as a Function of Psychological Openness." *Journal of Counseling Psychology* 14 (1967): 35-41.

Alexik, M., and Carkhuff, R. "The Effects of Manipulation of Client Depth of Self-Exploration upon High- and Low-Functioning Counselors." *Journal of Clinical Psychology* 23 (1967): 210-12.

Arnold, M. *Emotion and Personality,* 2 volumes. New York: Columbia University Press, 1960.

Ausubel, D. "The Use of Advance Organizers in the Learning and Retention of Meaningful Verbal Material." *Journal of Educational Psychology* 51 (1960): 267-72.

Bandura, A. *Principles of Behavior Modification,* New York: McGraw-Hill Book Co., 1969.

Bandura, A., and Whalen, C. "The Influence of Antecedent Reinforcement and Divergent Modeling Cues on Patterns of Self-Reward." *Journal of Personality and Social Psychology* 3 (1966): 373-82.

Branden, N. "Emotions and Values." *The Objectivist* 5 (May 1966): 1-9.

Cannon J., and Carkhuff, R. "Effects of Rater Level of Functioning and Experience upon the Discrimination of Facilitative Conditions." *Journal of Consulting and Clinical Psychology* 33 (1968): 189-94.

Carkhuff, R. *Helping and Human Relations,* volumes 1 and 2. New York: Holt, Rinehart & Winston, 1969.

Dreyfus, E. *Youth: Search For Meaning.* Columbus, Ohio: Charles E. Merrill Publishing Co., 1971.

Egan, G. *Encounter Group Processes for Interpersonal Growth.* Belmont, California: Wadsworth Publishing Co., 1970.

Ellis, A., "A Humanistic Approach to Psychotherapy." *The Humanist* 2 (1970): 32-37.

————. "Objectivism, The New Religion: Part II." *Rational Living* 3 (1968): 12-19.

————. "The Rational-Emotive Encounter Group." In *Encounter: Theory and Practice of Encounter Groups,* edited by A. Burton, pp. 112-27. San Francisco: Jossey Bass, 1969.

————. *Reason and Emotion in Psychotherapy.* New York: Lyle Stuart, 1962.

————. "Teaching Emotional Education in the Classroom." *School Health Review* (November 1969): 10-13.

Ellis, A., and Harper, R. *A Guide to Rational Living.* Englewood Cliffs, New Jersey: Prentice-Hall, Inc., 1961; Hollywood, California: Wilshire Book Co., 1961.

Erikson, E. *Identity: Youth and Crises.* New York: W. W. Norton Co., 1968.

Farquhar, W., and Lowe, J. "A List of Ellis's Irrational Ideas." Unpublished paper, Michigan State University, 1968.

Frank, J. *Persuasion and Healing.* New York: Schocken Books, 1965.

Fromm, E. *The Art of Loving.* New York: Harper Calophon Books, 1962.

————. *Escape from Freedom.* New York: Holt, Rinehart, & Winston, 1941.

Fry, P. S. "Self-Imposed Delay of Gratification." *Journal of Counseling Psychology* 19 (May 1972): 234-37.

Goldstein, A.; Heller, K.; and Sechrest, L. *Psychotherapy and the Psychology of Behavior Change.* New York: John Wiley and Sons, 1966.

Guilford, J. *The Nature of Human Intelligence.* New York: McGraw-Hill Book Co., 1967.

Hartman, B. "Sixty Revealing Questions for Twenty Minutes." *Rational Living* 43 (1968): 7-8.

Inhelder, B., and Piaget, J. *The Growth of Logical Thinking from Childhood to Adolescence,* translated by Anne Parsons and Stanley Milgram. New York: Basic Books, Inc., 1958.

Jourard, S. *An Experimental Analysis of the Transparent Self.* New York: Wiley-Interscience, 1971.

Kelly, G. *The Psychology of Personal Constructs.* New York: W. W. Norton Co., 1955.

Kemp, C. "Influence of Dogmatism in Counseling." *Personnel and Guidance Journal* 39 (1961): 662-65.

Krumboltz, J., and Thoresen, C. "The Effect of Behavioral Counseling in Group and Individual Settings on Information Seeking Behavior." *Journal of Counseling Psychology* 11 (1964): 324-33.

Lazarus, A. "New Techniques for Behavioral Change." *Rational Living* 6 (1971): 3-7.

Lindsley, D. "Psychophysiology and Motivation." *Nebraska Symposium on Motivation,* edited by M. R. June, pp. 44-105. Lincoln: University of Nebraska Press, 1957.

Lowen, A. "Bio-Energetic Group Therapy." In *Group Therapy Today,* edited by H. M. Rutenbeck, pp. 279-90. New York: Atherton Press, 1969.

Maslow, A. *Toward a Psychology of Being.* New York: Van Nostrand Co., 1962.

Maultsby, M. "Rational-Emotive Imagery. "*Rational Living* 6 (1971): 16-23.

_____. "Routine Tape Recorder Use in RET." *Rational Living* 5 (1969): 8-23.

_____. "Systematic Homework in Written Psychotherapy." *Rational Living* 6 (1971): 16-23.

Mooney, R. "A Conceptual Model for Integrating Four Approaches to the Identification of Creative Talent." In *Scientific Creativity: Its Recognition and Development,* edited by C. Taylor and F. Barron. New York: John Wiley Sons, 1963.

Morustakas, C. *Lonliness.* Englewood Cliffs, New Jersey: Prentice Hall, Inc. 1961.

Perls, F. *Gestalt Therapy Verbatim.* Lafayette, California: Real People Press, 1969.

Piaget, J. *The Origins of Intelligence in Children.* New York: W. W. Norton Co., 1963.

Premack, D. "Reinforcement Theory." In *Nebraska Symposium on Motivation,* edited by David Levine, pp. 123-88. Lincoln: University of Nebraska Press, 1965.

Quaranta, J. "Conceptual Framework for Career Development Programming." In *Guidance for Planning and Evaluative Career Development,* edited by R. McCormick and J. Wigtil. Project sponsored by the Division of Guidance and Testing. Columbus: Ohio Department of Education, 1971.

Robison, F. *Effective Study Skills.* New York: Harper and Row, 1946.

Rogers, C.R. "The Characteristics of the Helping Relationships." *Personnel and Guidance Journal* 31 (1958): 6-16.

_____. "The Interpersonal Relationship: The Core of Guidance." *Harvard Educational Review* 32 (1962): 416-29.

Sartre, J. *Being and Nothingness: An Essay on Phenomenological Ontology*, translated by Hazel Barner. New York: Philosophical Library, 1956.

Schutz, W.C. *Here Comes Everybody*, New York: Harper & Row, 1971.

Tosi, D. "Dogmatism within the Counselor-Client Dyad." *Journal of Counseling Psychology* 17 (1970): 284-88.

_____. "On the Continuation of Title III Projects following Termination of Funding: An Interpersonal Model." Paper presented to the Michigan State Department of Education, Division of Title III, 1971.

Tosi, D., and Liggit. "Rational Emotive Guidance in the Junior High School." Research project in progress, 1973.

_____. "A Factor Analysis of the Personal Orientation Inventory." *Journal of Humanistic Psychology* (Spring 1972): 86-93.

Tosi, D.; Briggs, R.D.; and Morley, R.M. "Study Habit Modification and Its Effect on Academic Performance: A Behavioral Approach." *The Journal of Educational Research* 6 (1971): 8.

Truax, C. "Reinforcement and Nonreinforcement in Rogerian Psychotherapy." *Journal of Abnormal Psychiatry* 71 (1966): 1-9.

VanderVeen, F. "The Perception by Clients and by Judges of the Conditions Offered by the Therapist in the Therapy Relationship." *Psychiatric Institute Bulletin* 1 (1961).

Wolfe, J. "How Integrative is Integrative Therapy? *The Counseling Psychologist* 2-3 (1972): 42-49.

Wolpe, J. *Psychotherapy by Reciprocal Inhibition*. Palo Alto, California: Stanford University Press, 1966.

index

159

other publications in the counseling youth series edited by herman peters

youth: search for meaning
edward a. dreyfus

youth: critical issues
marvin powell

counseling techniques with youth
frank h. krause and donald e. hendrickson

for those who care: ways of relating to youth
charles l. thompson and william a. poppen

youth: myths and realities
richard r. stevic and robert h. rossberg

experimenting with living: pros and cons
roger f. aubrey

counseling the culturally different black youth
elsie j. smith

youth: self-concept and behavior
james c. hansen and peter e. maynard

youth: new perspectives on old dimensions
james j. muro

charles e. merrill publishing company
a bell & howell company
columbus, ohio 43216

8877